Radio/Phone Consultation

Identify: Unit #	Your Name
Patient Age	Sex
Chief Complaint (onset, duration, etc.)	
LOC	Level of Distress
Signs and Symptoms	
Heart Rate	BP
Respirations	SpO_2%
Skin	Pupils
Lung Sounds	ECG
Past Medical HX	
Medications	
Allergies	
Emergency Care	
Physician	
ETA	En Route
Time	Other

Rapid Sequence Intubation

Prepare equipment (IV, ECG, oximeter, BVM, suction, ETT); CO_2 detector; backup airway

↓

Spinal motion restriction, if indicated

↓

Preoxygenate with 100% O_2; apply and maintain cricoid pressure

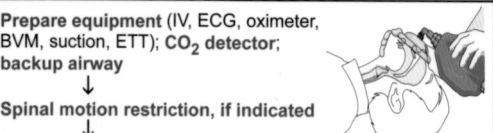

Place patient in sniff position; hyperventilate with O_2

↓

Give sedative
· Midazolam 0.1–0.3 mg/kg IV/IO *OR:*
· Thiopental 1–3 mg/kg IV/IO *OR:*
· Ketamine 1–2 mg/kg IV/IO *OR:*
· Etomidate 0.3 mg/kg IV/IO *OR:*
· Diazepam 0.2 mg/kg IV/IO
  (maximum 20 mg)

↓

If patient <2 years old, **consider Atropine** 0.02 mg/kg IV/IO (may block reflex bradycardia)

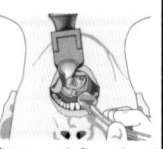

Lift tongue leftward and visualize vocal cords

↓

Give Succinylcholine 1–1.5 mg/kg IV/IO *OR:* Rocuronium 0.6–1.2 mg/kg IV/IO *OR:* Vecuronium 0.1 mg/kg IV/IO

↓

Intubate

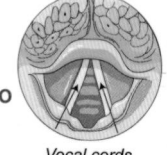

Vocal cords

↓

Inflate cuff; verify tube placement
· Check chest expansion
· Check lung sounds
· Fogging of tube
· Apply CO_2 detector
· Secure with ETT holder
  C-collar (if applicable)

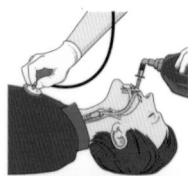

Insert ETT; inflate cuff; check breath sounds

King LT Airway

Contra—Patients <4 feet tall. Does not protect against aspiration.

1. **C-Spine immobilization**, as needed. Preoxygenate with 100% O_2. Apply water-based lube to distal tip and posterior aspect of tube.

Step 2

2. **Deflate cuff**. Open mouth, apply chin lift, **insert tip into side of mouth**.

3. **Advance tip behind tongue** while rotating tube to midline.

4. **Advance tube** until base of connector is aligned with teeth or gums.

5. **Inflate cuff** with air (use minimum volume necessary).

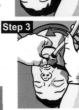
Step 3

Patient Size	LT Size	Cuff Vol
35–45 inches	Size 2	25–35 mL
41–51 inches	Size 2.5	30–40 mL
4–5 feet	Size 3	45–60 mL
5–6 feet	Size 4	60–80 mL
>6 feet	Size 5	70–90 mL

Step 4

6. **Attach bag-valve device**. While ventilating, gently withdraw tube until ventilation becomes easy.

7. **Adjust cuff inflation**, if necessary, to obtain a good seal.

Step 6

8. **Verify proper placement**
   - Check chest expansion and lung sounds
   - Apply CO_2 detector; oximeter
   - Secure with tape or tube holder
   - Reassess airway periodically

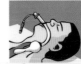

Trauma

Trauma Triage Chart

(See also, "Trauma Cardiac Arrest" in ACLS section)

MEASURE VITAL SIGNS AND LEVEL OF CONSCIOUSNESS

PHYSIOLOGICAL CRITERIA

Glasgow Coma Scale   < 14 or
Systolic blood pressure   < 90 or
Respiratory rate   < 10 or > 29 (< 20 in infant < one year)

YES	NO
Take to a trauma center. These patients should be transported preferentially to the highest level of care within the trauma system.	Assess anatomy of injury

ANATOMICAL CRITERIA

- All penetrating injuries to head, neck, torso, and extremities proximal to elbow and knee
- Flail chest
- Two or more proximal long-bone fractures
- Crushed, degloved, or mangled extremity
- Amputation proximal to wrist and ankle
- Pelvic fractures
- Open or depressed skull fracture
- Paralysis

YES	NO
Take to a trauma center. These patients should be transported preferentially to the highest level of care within the trauma system.	Assess mechanism of injury and evidence of high-energy impact

Go to next page

MECHANISM OF INJURY

Falls
- Adults: > 20 ft. (one story is equal to 10 ft.)
- Children: > 10 ft. or 2-3 times the height of the child

High-Risk Auto Crash
- Intrusion: > 12 in. occupant site; > 18 in. any site
- Ejection (partial or complete) from automobile
- Death in same passenger compartment
- Vehicle telemetry data consistent with high risk of injury

Auto vs Pedestrian/Bicyclist Thrown, Run Over, or with Significant (> 20 MPH) Impact

Motorcycle Crash > 20 MPH

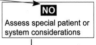

YES	**NO**
Transport to closest appropriate trauma center, which depending on the trauma system, need not be the highest level trauma center.	Assess special patient or system considerations

SPECIAL POPULATIONS (Cormorbidities)

Age
- Older Adults: Risk of injury death increases after age 55
- SBP < 110 might represent shock after 65 years
- Low impact mechanisms (e.g. ground level falls) may result in serious injuries
- Children: Should be triaged preferentially to pediatric-capable trauma centers

Anticoagulation and Bleeding Disorders

Burns
- Without other trauma mechanism: Triage to burn facility
- With trauma mechanism: Triage to trauma center

Time-Sensitive Extremity Injury

End-Stage Renal Disease Requiring Dialysis

Pregnancy > 20 Weeks

EMS Provider Judgment

YES	**NO**
Contact medical control and consider transport to a trauma center or a specific resource hospital.	Transport according to protocol

Rapid Triage

(For multiple patient scenes.)

Priority	Color	Condition	Notes
0	Black	Deceased	No care needed
1	Red	Immediate	Life threatening
2	Yellow	Urgent	Can delay up to 1 hour
3	Green	Delayed	Up to 3 hours

Priority 0—Deceased, No Care Needed

No pulse, no respirations (open airway first), obvious mortal wounds (e.g., decapitation).

Priority 1—Immediate Transport

Unconscious, disoriented, very confused, rapid respirations, weak irregular pulse, severe uncontrolled bleeding, other signs of shock (cold, clammy skin, low blood pressure, etc.).

Priority 2—Urgent, Can Delay Transport Up To 1 hour

Conscious, oriented, with any significant fracture or other significant injury, but without signs of shock.

Priority 3—Delayed Transport Up To 3 hours

Walking wounded, CAO x3, minor injuries.

NOTE: Assessment of patients should be <15 seconds each. (Have someone else control bleeding during your survey.)
* All unconscious patients are Priority 1—Immediate
* "Walking wounded" are usually GREEN—Priority 3
* All pulseless patients are BLACK—Priority 0

Mentation/LOC Assessment

A—Alert	Able to answer questions.	
V—Verbal	Responds to verbal stimuli.	
P—Pain	Responds only to pain stimuli. Protect airway.	
U—Unconscious	Protect airway	

Multiple Patients

1. Strategically park vehicle and stay in one place

2. **Establish Command**, and identify yourself as Command to dispatch (use a calm, clear voice)

3. **Size up the scene** and advise dispatch of:
   - Exact location and type of incident
   - Estimated number and severity of patients
   - Any hazardous conditions
   - The best routes of access to the scene
   - The location of the command post

4. Designate an EMT to perform rapid triage (see *Trauma section, Rapid Triage,* for more contraindications), tag and number multiple patients ("Immediate," "**Urgent**," "Delayed")

5. **Order resources** (Fire, Police, Ambulances, HazMat, Extrication, Air Units, Tow vehicles, Buses, etc.)

6. Set up staging areas (clearly state the location of staging/assembly areas, and think of access and egress)

7. **Coordinate access** of incoming units to the scene

8. **Assign patients** to incoming medical units

9. Maintain communications with On-Line Medical Control (OLMC)

10. **Keep patient log** indicating patient number, name, severity, treating and transporting units, medical interventions, and destination hospitals

Mass Casualty Incident

NOTE: Use Multiple Patient guidelines above, and the following ICS groups.

Medical Branch Director

- Reports to IC
- Responsible for overall medical direction/coordination
- Orders additional medical resources
- Serves as a resource for group supervisors

Triage Group Supervisor

- Estimates number and severity of patients
- Establishes tagging and extrication teams
- Establishes triage areas, if necessary
- Maintains rapid and orderly flow of patients to treatment areas

Treatment Area Group Supervisor

- Secures treatment areas, identifies equipment needs
- Clearly marks Treatment Areas for "Immediate," "**Urgent**," "Delayed"
- Establishes treatment teams when resources allow
- Identifies order of patient transport

Transportation Group Supervisor

- Establishes Patient Loading Zone (near Treatment Area)
- Assigns patients to ambulances, supervises actual loading
- Relays Unit number, severity and number of patients to Communications Group Supervisor

Communications Group Supervisor

- Communicates with On-line Medical Control (OLMC) to identify receiving hospitals
- Maintains patient log
- Receives information from Transportation Group
- Coordinates patient destinations to avoid overloading the closest hospitals

Abbreviations Used In This Section

HX—History, Signs, and Symptoms
PRN -- if needed
Key Symptoms and Findings (green text)
➕—**Prehospital Treatment** (blue text with yellow background)
Cautions—Contraindications or Precautions (red text)

Trauma—Abdominal

HX—Mechanism of injury, associated trauma, penetrating vs. blunt injury? Suspect internal hemorrhage. **Guarding, distension, rigidity, hypotension, pallor, bruising?**
➕—Vitals, O_2 PRN, IV, treat for shock, transport.

Trauma—Burns

HX—Airway burns (red mouth, persistent wheezing, cough, hoarseness, dyspnea)? Was patient in enclosed space? How long? Did patient lose consciousness? Was there an explosion? Toxic fumes? Hx cardiac or lung disease? Estimate % of burns and depth. Other trauma?

NOTE: Significant burns = blistered or charred areas, or burns of the hands, feet, face, airway, genitalia.

➕ —**Stop the burning**: Extinguish clothing if smoldering.
- Remove clothing, if not adhered to skin; remove jewelry.
- Vitals, give high flow O_2, assist ventilations if needed.
- ❖ **Superficial and Deep Superficial Burns**: If <20%, apply wet dressings.
- ❖ **Moderate to Severe Burns**: Cover with dry sterile dressing (DSD) and/or burn sheet. Leave blisters intact. Start large bore IV, treat for shock or % burn. Monitor ECG.
- ❖ **Chemical Burns**: Brush off any dry chemical then flush with copious amounts of water or saline.
  For lime: Brush off excess, then flush; For phosphorus: Use **copious** amounts of water.
- ❖ **Electrical Burns**: Apply DSD to entry and exit wounds. Start large bore IV, titrate for shock. Monitor ECG—treat dysrhythmias per ACLS.

Cautions—Consider child abuse in pediatric patients.

WARNING: Do not apply ointments to burns. Avoid starting IV in burned area if possible. Consider carbon monoxide (CO) poisoning. Conventional pulse oximetry not accurate with CO.

Burn Chart

NOTE: Count only second degree and third degree burns.

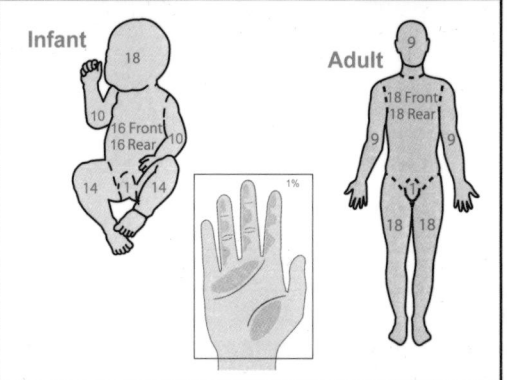

Prehospital IV Fluid Resuscitation

- < 30 min. from ED, no fluid needed
- > 30 min. transport, Lactated Ringer's:
  - > 14 yo – 500 mL/hour
  - 6–13 yo – 250 mL/hour
  - < 5 yo – 125 mL/hour

NOTE: Major burns should be treated in a burn center, including: ≥25% body surface; hands, feet, face, or perineum; electrical burns; inhalation burns; other injuries; or severe pre-existing medical problems. Burns require pain management.

Trauma—Cardiac Arrest
(See ACLS section, Trauma Cardiac Arrest algorithm)

NOTE: Rapid extrication and transport immediately.

✚—Secure airway, do CPR (shock VF), O_2, IVs en route. Splint fractures en route.

Trauma—Chest

NOTE: Suspect cardiac, pulmonary, or great vessel trauma.

✚—Secure airway, high flow O_2, intubate if necessary and assist ventilations. Open chest wound: cover with occlusive dressing. Look for exit wounds. Tension pneumothorax: evaluate and decompress. Impaled objects: stabilize in place. Do not delay transport if patient is unstable. Consider IV fluids for shock (2 large bore IVs), monitor ECG, vitals. Full spinal immobilization.

Cautions—Consider other causes for respiratory distress.

Trauma—Crush Injury with Entrapment

NOTE: While crushed, the patient's BP, HR, and RR may appear normal. Sudden release can cause reperfusion syndrome (Crush Syndrome).

✚—Give patient dust mask or O_2 mask (humidified best), treat for hypothermia, start IV fluids BEFORE crush mechanism lifted, especially if crushed >4 hours. If IV fluids not possible, consider short-term use of tourniquet on affected limb until IV hydration initiated. Safety glasses and noise protection, as needed.

PREVENT:
- **Hypotension**: a result of third spacing and hemorrhage
- **Renal failure**: IV fluids, mannitol, dialysis
- **Acidosis**: sodium bicarbonate
- **Hyperkalemia/hypocalcemia**: consider calcium, insulin, D50 and kayexalate with sorbitol
- **Cardiac arrhythmia**: treat accordingly to ACLS guidelines; monitor for pain, pallor, parasthesias, pain with passive movement, pulselessness

CAUTION: If >1 hour of crush, do not release crushing mechanism until ready.

Trauma—Head

✚—Secure airway while providing spinal motion restriction. Control bleeding with direct pressure. Do not stop bleeding from nose, ears if CSF leak is suspected, O_2 PRN (TKO unless patient is in shock). Monitor vitals and neuro status. ECG, oximetry; consider intubation and ventilation if GCS ≤8. Hyperventilate to ETCO$_2$ of 30–35. Elevate HOB 15°–30°.

Cautions—Always suspect C-spine injury in the head injury patient. Assess and document LOC changes. Be alert for airway problems and seizures. Restlessness and or agitation can be due to hypoxia or hypoglycemia. Check Chemstrip®.

Glasgow Coma Scale

NOTE: Patient with a score of 3–8 is in a coma and needs ventilatory support.

Eye Opening

INFANT			CHILD/ADULT
4	Spontaneously	Spontaneously	4
3	To speech	To command	3
2	To pain	To pain	2
1	No response	No response	1

Best Verbal Response

5	Coos, babbles	Oriented	5
4	Irritable cries	Confused	4
3	Cries to pain	Inappropriate words	3
2	Moans, grunts	Incomprehensible	2
1	No response	No response	1

Best Motor Response

6	Spontaneous	Obeys commands	6
5	Localizes pain	Localizes pain	5
4	Withdraws from pain	Withdraws from pain	4
3	Flexion (decorticate)	Flexion (decorticate)	3
2	Extension (decerebrate)	Extension (decereb.)	2
1	No response	No response	1

____ = Total →(GCS ≤8? →Intubate!) ← Total = ____

Trauma

Trauma—Spinal Injury

HX—MOI, helmet worn? Suspect C-spine injury with head or neck trauma, and with multi-system trauma, or diving/drowning. Altered mental status? Is there paralysis, weakness, numbness, tingling? Spinal pain with or without movement, point tenderness, deformity, or guarding?

✚—Keep airway open. Consider nasopharyngeal airway. Splint neck with C-collar and spinal motion restriction. Move the patient as a unit and only as necessary. Give O$_2$ PRN, Start large bore IV. Vitals. **Place patient in Trauma System**.

Cautions—Be prepared to suction and/or move the patient as a unit while immobilized. Consider internal bleeding.

Spinal Innervation

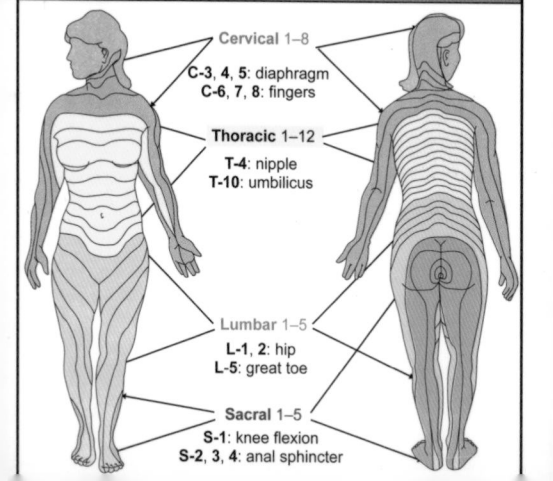

Cervical 1–8

C-3, 4, 5: diaphragm
C-6, 7, 8: fingers

Thoracic 1–12

T-4: nipple
T-10: umbilicus

Lumbar 1–5

L-1, 2: hip
L-5: great toe

Sacral 1–5

S-1: knee flexion
S-2, 3, 4: anal sphincter

ACLS Algorithms

NOTE: ECGs illustrated in this guide are for reference only and should not be interpreted as exact.

NOTE: Not all patients require the treatment indicated by these algorithms. These algorithms assume that you have assessed the patient, started CPR where indicated, and performed reassessment after each treatment. These algorithms also do not exclude other appropriate interventions which may be warranted by the patient's condition.
Treat the patient, not the ECG.

Notes

Cardiac Arrest

Shout for help, begin CPR (30:2, push hard and fast at 100–120 min. minimize interruptions), give O_2, attach ECG.

YES ⇦ Shockable Rhythm? ⇨ **NO**

VF or VT	Asystole/PEA

VF or VT

⇩

✎ **Defibrillate 120 J–200 J** Biphasic (or 360 J monophasic, or AED)

⇩

Continue CPR immediately x2 minutes. Start IV/IO.

⇩

VF/VT?

⇩

✎ **Defibrillate**
Continue CPR x2 minutes.
Epinephrine 1 mg IV/IO, repeat every 3–5 minutes
Consider advanced airway (ET Tube, supraglottic airway)
Ventilate 10 breaths/minute with continuous compressions.

Use waveform capnography: If $PETCO_2$ <10, improve CPR.

⇩

VF/VT?

⇩

✎ **Defibrillate**
Continue CPR x2 minutes.
Amiodarone 300 mg IV/IO, (may repeat once 150 mg in 5 minutes)
Consider Reversible Causes.❖

⇩

If ROSC (pulse, BP, $PETCO_2$ ≥40 mm Hg), see *ROSC algorithm*, next page.

Asystole/PEA

⇩

Continue CPR immediately x2 minutes. Start IV/IO.
Epinephrine 1 mg IV/IO, repeat every 3–5 minutes **Consider advanced airway** (ET Tube, supraglottic airway)
Ventilate 10 breaths/min. with continuous compressions.

Use waveform capnography: If $PETCO_2$ <10, improve CPR.

⇩

Asystole/PEA?

⇩

Continue CPR x2 minutes.
Consider Reversible Causes.❖

⇩

If ROSC (pulse, BP, $PETCO_2$ ≥40 mm Hg), see *ROSC algorithm*, next page.

❖**Reversible Causes:**
• Hypoxia
• Hypovolemia
• Acidosis
• Hyper/Hypokalemia
• Hypothermia
• Coronary Thrombosis
• Cardiac Tamponade
• Tension Pneumothorax
• Toxins

Return of Spontaneous Circulation: Post Cardiac Arrest Care

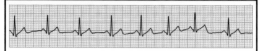

Optimize Ventilation/Oxygenation
(start at 10 breaths per minute, but *do not hyperventilate*)
Goal: PETCO$_2$ 35–40 mm Hg.
Use minimum amount of FiO$_2$ to keep SaO$_2$ ≥94%
Consider waveform capnography
⇩
Keep blood pressure ≥90 mm Hg (or MAP ≥65)
IV fluid bolus: 1–2 Liter(s) NS or RL

Consider vasopressor infusion
Epinephrine: 0.1–0.5 mcg/kg/minute
Dopamine: 5–10 mcg/kg/minute
Norepinephrine: 0.1–0.5 mcg/kg/minute

Consider Reversible Causes❖
Monitor ECG, obtain 12-lead ECG
⇩
Follows commands?
(if not, consider targeted temperature management)
⇩
STEMI or High suspicion AMI?
⇩
Coronary reperfusion (PCI)
Advanced critical care

❖Reversible Causes:
- Hypoxia
- Acidosis
- Hypovolemia
- Toxins
- Coronary Thrombosis
- Cardiac Tamponade
- Hyper/Hypokalemia
- Hypothermia
- Pulmonary Thrombosis
- Tension Pneumothorax

ACLS

Field Determination of Death

EMS Clinical Exam for Death:
- Time of assessment (this is the time of death)
- No response to verbal or tactile stimulation
- No pupillary light reflex (pupils fixed and dilated)
- Absence of breath sounds
- Absence of heart sounds
- AED or EKG = no signs of life

EMS Death Documentation:
- Describe your exam
- Location/position where found
- Physical condition of body
- Significant medical Hx or trauma
- Conditions precluding resuscitation
- Any medical control contact
- Person body left in custody of

Tips:
- Following field termination of resuscitation, observe patient for at least 10 minutes for autoresuscitation (return of vital signs)
- Isolated fatal injuries may be candidates for organ donation
- Some patients underwater for less than 2 hours have survived (never > 2 hours)
- Beware of hypothermia, cannot declare death until core temp > 90°F

Bradycardia

(HR <50/minute with serious S/Sx: shock, hypotension, altered mental status, ischemic chest pain, acute heart failure.)

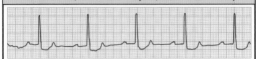

Assess C-A-B, maintain airway, give O_2 PRN, assist breathing if needed. Attach pulse oximeter, BP cuff, 12-lead ECG, start IV/IO.

Consider and Treat Reversible Causes

⇩

Atropine 0.5 mg IV/IO every 3–5 minutes, maximum: 3 mg (Do not delay TCP while starting IV, or waiting for Atropine to work*.) *If ineffective:*

⇩

Transcutaneous Pacing (verify capture and perfusion; use sedation as needed) *OR:*
Dopamine 2–20 mcg/kg per minute, *OR:*
Epinephrine 2–10 mcg per minute

⇩

Consider expert consult; prepare for transvenous pacer

⇩

Cardiac Arrest? —See *ACLS section, Cardiac Arrest Algorithm*

❖Reversible Causes:
- Hypoxia
- Acidosis
- Hypovolemia
- Toxins
- Coronary Thrombosis
- Cardiac Tamponade
- Hyper/Hypokalemia
- Hypothermia
- Pulmonary Thrombosis
- Tension Pneumothorax

*Atropine may not work for transplanted hearts, Mobitz (Type II) AV Block or third degree AV Block with IVR.

—Begin pacing, and/or catecholamine infusion.

UNSYMPTOMATIC BRADYCARDIA?
— NOT Type II (Mobitz) second degree or third degree AV heart block?

⇩

Observe

Tachycardias

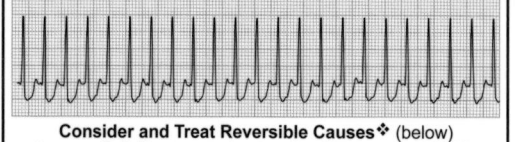

Consider and Treat Reversible Causes ❖ (below)
Assess C-A-B, secure airway, give O$_2$ PRN, **start IV/IO,**
check BP, apply Oximeter, get 12-lead ECG

Is Patient Unstable?	Stable?

(Serious S/Sx must be related to the tachycardia:
HR ≥150, ischemic chest pain, dyspnea, ↓LOC,
↓BP, shock, heart failure.)

Go to next
page

✐ **Immediate Synchronized Cardioversion**
(for narrow QRS, consider Adenosine 6 mg, rapid IVP
(flush with NS, may repeat with 12 mg IVP); **also
consider sedation,** but do not delay cardioversion)
Initial Energy Doses: (if unsuccessful, increase
doses in a stepwise fashion.)
Narrow QRS, Regular: 50 J–100 J
Narrow QRS, Irregular: 120 J–200 J biphasic,
(or 200 J monophasic)
Wide QRS, Regular: 100 J
Wide QRS, Irregular: defibrillate with 120 J–200 J
biphasic, (or 360 J monophasic)

Synchronize Markers

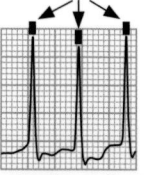

Pad/paddle placement
for synchronized
cardioversion

Synchronize on R wave

Stable Patient, Wide QRS (≥0.12 seconds)	Stable Patient, Narrow QRS (<0.12 second)
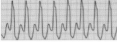	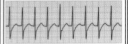

Stable Patient, Wide QRS (≥0.12 seconds)

- 12-lead ECG
- Start IV
- **Consider Adenosine 6 mg IVP** (for regular, monomorphic rhythm) flush with saline, may repeat 12 mg IVP
- **Consider antiarrhythmic:**
  Either:

Procainamide
20–50 mg/minute IV until rhythm converts, QRS widens by 50%, hypotension, or maximum dose 17 mg/kg. Avoid if CHF or prolonged QT. Drip 1–4 mg/minute.
OR:

Amiodarone 150 mg IV over 10 minutes. May repeat, (maximum dose: 2.2 gm IV/24 hours). Drip 1 mg/minute
OR:

Sotalol 1.5 mg/kg IV over 5 min. Avoid if prolonged QT.
- **Consult with expert**

For Polymorphic VT (Torsades), give magnesium sulfate 2 gms IV over 1-2 minutes.

Stable Patient, Narrow QRS (<0.12 second)

- 12-lead ECG
- Start IV
- Vagal maneuvers*
- **Adenosine 6 mg IVP** (for regular rhythm) flush with saline, may repeat 12 mg IVP
  Either:
- **Calcium blocker** (choose one:)
Verapamil 2.5–5 mg IV over 2–3 minutes. May repeat 5–10 mg. Maximum 30 mg.
Diltiazem 0.25 mg/kg IV over 2 minutes. May repeat 0.35 mg/kg.
  OR:
- **Beta blocker** (choose one:)
Metoprolol 5 mg IV over 2–5 minutes. May repeat. Maximum 15 mg.
Atenolol 5 mg IV over 5 minutes. May repeat once.
Propranolol 1–3 mg IV slowly over 2–5 minutes.
Esmolol 250–500 mcg/kg x1 minute.
- **Consult with expert**

*Carotid sinus massage is contraindicated in patients with carotid bruits. Avoid ice application to face, if patient has ischemic heart disease.

Asthma Cardiac Arrest

Use standard ACLS Guidelines
Endotracheal intubation via RSI
(use largest ET tube possible; monitor waveform capnography)

⇩

To reduce hyperinflation, hypotension, and risk of tension pneumothorax, consider:
- **Ventilate with a slower respiratory rate**
- **Smaller tidal volume (6–8 mL/kg)**
- **Shorter inspiratory time (80–100 mL/minute)**
- **Longer expiratory time (I/E 1:4 or 1:5)**

⇩

**Continue inhaled beta$_2$ agonist (albuterol)
via ET tube**
Evaluate for tension pneumothorax

⇩

Consider corticosteroids

⇩

Consult with expert

⇩

**Consider: brief disconnect from BVM and
press on chest wall during exhalation
to relieve air trapping**

⇩

If the patient suddenly deteriorates

⇩

DOPE:
- **Displacement of ETT**
- **Obstruction of tube**
- **Pneumothorax**
- **Equipment failure**
- **Evaluate for Auto-PEEP**

Cardiac Arrest During PCI

- **Consider mechanical CPR**
- **Consider emergency cardiopulmonary bypass**
- **Consider Cough CPR**
- **Consider intracoronary verapamil for reperfusion induced Ventricular Tachycardia**

Cardiac Tamponade Cardiac Arrest

- Emergency pericardiocentesis/pericardial window
- **Consider emergency department thoracotomy**

Drowning Cardiac Arrest

- Begin rescue breathing ASAP
- **Start CPR with A-B-C** (Airway and Breathing first)
- **Anticipate vomiting** (have suction ready)
- **Attach AED** (dry chest off with towel)
- **Check for hypothermia**
- Use Standard BLS and ACLS

Electrocution Cardiac Arrest

(Respiratory arrest is common)

- Is the scene safe?
- Triage patients and treat those with respiratory arrest or cardiac arrest first
- **Start CPR**
- **Stabilize the cervical spine**
- **Attach AED**
- **Remove smoldering clothing**
- **Check for trauma**
- **Large bore IV for rapid fluid administration**
- **Consider early intubation for airway burns**
- Use Standard BLS and ACLS

24

Electrolyte Imbalance Cardiac Arrest

Hyperkalemia:

Wide QRS, peaked
T waves, IVR,
heart block, VF

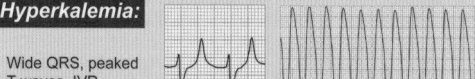

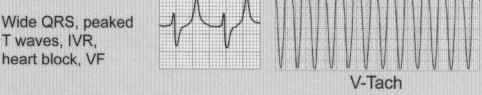

V-Tach

Calcium chloride 10% 500–1,000 mg IV/IO (5–10 mL) over
2–5 minutes [or calcium gluconate 10% 15–30 mL over
2–5 minutes].
Sodium bicarbonate 50 mEq IV/IO over 5 minutes [may repeat in 15
minutes]
**Dextrose 25 grams (50 mL of D50) IV/IO + Regular Insulin
10 Units IV/IO** over 15–30 minutes
Albuterol 10–20 mg nebulized over 15 minutes
Furosemide 40–80 mg IV/IO

Hypokalemia: Use Standard BLS and ACLS

Long QT interval, flat T waves, U wave

Hypermagnesemia:

Stop magnesium infusion
Consider: Calcium chloride 10% 500–1,000 mg IV/IO
(5–10 mL) over 2–5 minutes [or calcium gluconate 10%
15–30 mL over 2–5 minutes]

Signs and symptoms: **muscle weakness, paralysis, drowsiness,
confusion**
Severe: **bradycardia, hypoventilation, cardiac arrhythmias**

Hypomagnesemia: Magnesium sulfate 1–2 grams IV/IO

Pulmonary Embolism Cardiac Arrest

(Pulseless electrical activity is common)
- Standard BLS and ACLS
- **Emergency echocardiography**
- **Fibrinolytic for presumed PE**
- Consult expert
- **Consider percutaneous mechanical thrombectomy or surgical embolectomy**

Trauma Cardiac Arrest

Consider Reversible Causes✥ (below)
- Stabilize cervical spine
- **Jaw thrust to open airway**
- **Direct pressure for hemorrhage**
- Standard CPR and defibrillation
- **Use advanced airway if BVM inadequate** (consider cricothyrotomy if ventilation impossible)
- **Administer IV fluids** for hypovolemia
- Consider resuscitative thoracotomy

✥Reversible Causes:
- Hypoxia
- Acidosis
- Hypovolemia
- Toxins
- Coronary Thrombosis
- Cardiac Tamponade
- Hyper/Hypokalemia
- Hypothermia
- Pulmonary Thrombosis
- Tension Pneumothorax

"Commotio Cordis": a blow to the anterior chest causing VF
- Prompt CPR and defibrillation
- Standard BLS and ACLS

Hypothermia

- Remove wet clothing and stop heat loss (cover with blankets and insulating equipment: give oxygen per local protocol)
- Keep patient horizontal
- Move patient gently, if possible; do not jostle
- Monitor core temperature and cardiac rhythm
- Treat underlying causes (drug overdose, alcohol, trauma, etc.) simultaneously with resuscitation
- Check responsiveness, breathing, pulse

If Pulse and Breathing	No Pulse/Apneic
34°C–36°C **93°F–97°F** (MILD hypothermia) Passive rewarming	Start CPR, Ventilate **Defibrillate VF/VT** **Biphasic: 120 J–200 J** OR: **Monophasic 360 J** **Resume CPR Immediately** [Consider further defibrillation attempts for VF/VT] See *ACLS section, Cardiac Arrest algorithm.*
30°C–34°C **86°F–93°F** (MODERATE hypothermia) Active external rewarming **forced-air rewarming**	Intubate, ventilate with warm, humid oxygen (42°C–46°C) **Start IV/IO, administer warm normal saline (43°C)** [Consider epinephrine 1 mg IV every 3–5 minutes]
<30°C <86°F (SEVERE hypothermia) Core rewarming (cardiopulmonary bypass, thoracic cavity warm water lavage, extracorporeal blood warming with partial bypass)	⇩ Continue CPR, **Transport to ED, start core rewarming when feasible. Continue resuscitation until patient is rewarmed.**
Adjunctive rewarming: • Warm IV fluids (43°C) • Warm, humid O$_2$ (42°C–46°C) • Peritoneal lavage • Extracorporeal rewarming • Esophageal rewarming tubes • Endovascular rewarming	⇩ After ROSC, rewarm patient to 32°C–34°C (90°F–93°F), or to normal body temperature.

Stemi Fibrinolytic Protocol
"Time is muscle"

"Door-to-Drug" time should be <30 minutes.

- **S/S**: Cx pain >15 minute, but <12 hours.
- **Get Stat 12-lead ECG.** (Must show ST elevation, or new LBBB.)
- **ECG and other findings consistent with AMI.**
- **Give**: O_2, **NTG, Morphine, ASA** (if no contraindications).
- **Start 2 IVs** (but do not delay transport).
- **Systolic/diastolic BP**: Right arm ___/___ Left arm ___/___.
- **Complete Fibrinolytic Checklist** (all should be "No"):
  - ❏ Systolic BP >180–200 mm Hg
  - ❏ Diastolic BP >100–110 mm Hg
  - ❏ Right arm vs. left arm BP difference >15 mm Hg
  - ❏ Stroke >3 hours or <3 months
  - ❏ Hx Structural CNS Disease
  - ❏ Head/Facial Trauma within 3 weeks
  - ❏ Major trauma, GI/GU bleed, or surgery within 4 weeks
  - ❏ On blood thinners; bleeding/clotting problems
  - ❏ Pregnancy
  - ❏ History intracranial hemorrhage
  - ❏ Advanced cancer, severe liver/renal disease

High-Risk Profile/Indications for Transfer:

(if any are checked, consider transport to a hospital capable of angiography and revascularization)

- ❏ Heart rate ≥100 bpm and SBP ≤100 mm Hg
- ❏ Pulmonary edema (rales)
- ❏ Signs of shock
- ❏ Received CPR
- ❏ Contraindications to fibrinolytics

If no contraindications and Dx of AMI is confirmed:

Administer fibrinolytic. Also consider: **anticoagulants**, and **standard ACS treatments**. *Signs of reperfusion include:* pain relief, ST-segment normalization, reperfusion dysrhythmias, resolution of conduction block, early cardiac marker peak.

3-Lead and MCL₁ Electrode Placement

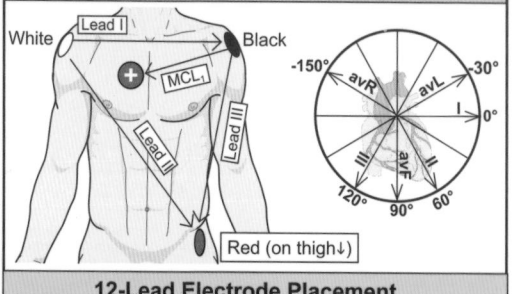

12-Lead Electrode Placement

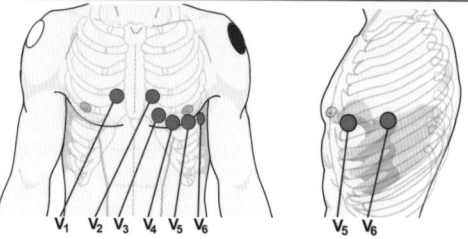

V₁: 4th interspace, just to the right of the sternum
V₂: 4th interspace, just to the left of the sternum
V₃: halfway between V₂ and V₄
V₄: 5th intercostal space, midclavicular line
V₅: anterior-axillary line, horizontal with V₄
V₆: mid-axillary line, horizontal with V₄
MCL₁: red lead on V₁, black lead on left arm—monitor lead III
MCL₆: red lead on V₆, white lead on right arm—monitor lead II
MC₄R: red lead on 5th ICS right mid-clavicular line, black lead on left arm—monitor lead III

Cardiac Arrest Rhythms

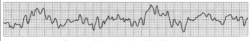

Coarse Ventricular Fibrillation
(Note the chaotic, irregular electrical activity) **Treatment:** Shock

Fine Ventricular Fibrillation
(Note the low-amplitude, irregular electrical activity)
Treatment: Shock

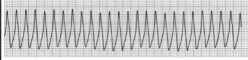

Ventricular Tachycardia
(Note the rapid, wide complexes) **Treatment:** Shock if no pulse

Asystole
(Note the absence of electrical activity) **Treatment:** Perform CPR

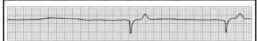

Pulseless Electrical Activity (PEA)
(Any organized ECG rhythm with no pulse)
Treatment: Perform CPR

Other Common ECG Rhythms

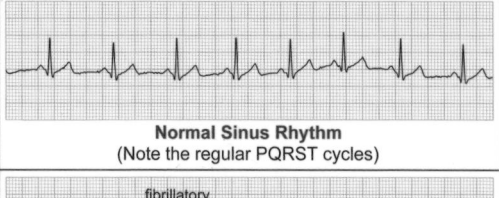

Normal Sinus Rhythm
(Note the regular PQRST cycles)

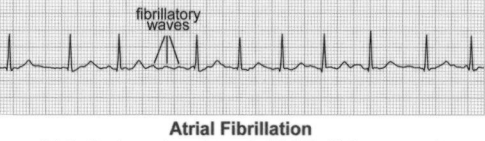

fibrillatory waves

Atrial Fibrillation
(Note the irregular rate and atrial fibrillatory waves)

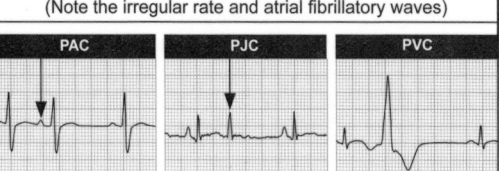

PAC	PJC	PVC
(normal QRS complex; different P wave)	(normal QRS complex; inverted or no P wave)	(wide, bizarre complex; no P wave)

Premature Atrial, Junctional, and Ventricular Complexes

Other Common ECG Rhythms

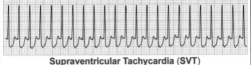

Supraventricular Tachycardia (SVT)
(Note the rapid, narrow QRS complexes)

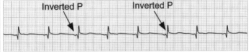

Inverted P   Inverted P

Junctional Rhythm
(Normal QRS complexes; inverted, or no P waves)

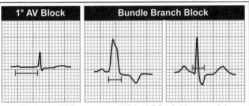

1° AV Block | **Bundle Branch Block**

(Prolonged PR Interval >0.20 seconds) | (Wide QRS >0.12 seconds)

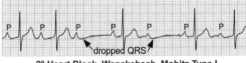

P   P   P   P   P   P   P

dropped QRS

2° Heart Block, Wenckebach, Mobitz Type I
(The PR interval lengthens, resulting in a dropped QRS)

Other Common ECG Rhythms

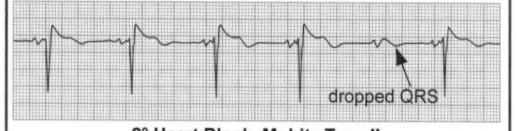

2° Heart Block, Mobitz Type II
(The PR interval does not lengthen; but a QRS is dropped)

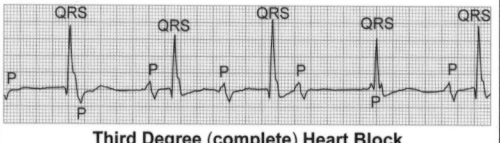

Third Degree (complete) Heart Block
(The P waves are dissociated from the QRS complexes)

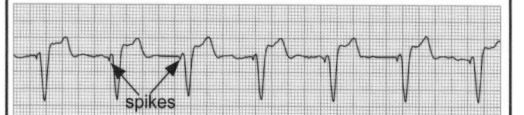

Electronic Ventricular Pacemaker
(Note the pacer spikes before each QRS)

Rapid Interpretation—-12-Lead ECG

❶ **Identify the rhythm**. If supraventricular (Sinus Rhythm, Atrial Fibrillation, Atrial Tachycardia, Atrial Flutter):

❷ **Rule out LBBB** (QRS >0.12 seconds; and R–R' in I, or V_5, or V_6).
LBBB confounds the Dx of AMI/ACS (unless it is new-onset LBBB).

LBBB
I, V_5, V_6

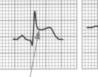

❸ If no LBBB, **check for**
ST segment elevation, *OR*
ST depression with T wave inversion, *OR* pathologic Q waves.

ST elevation	T wave inversion	Wide or deep QS

❹ Means acute MI | **May mean myocardial ischemia**, or impending MI | **Means infarction**

❺ **Rule out other confounders**: WPW (mimics infarct, BBB), pericarditis (mimics MI), digoxin (depresses STs), LVH (depresses STs, inverts T)

❻ **Identify location of infarct and consider appropriate treatments** (MONA, PCI [or fibrinolytic], nitrate infusion, heparin, GP IIb, IIIa inhibitor, beta blockers, antiarrhythmic, etc.)

Normal 12-Lead ECG

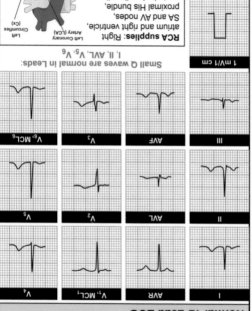

Small Q waves are normal in leads: I, II, AVL, V5, V6

RCA supplies: Right atrium and right ventricle, SA and AV nodes, proximal His bundle, posterior hemibundle.

LCA supplies: Left atrium and left ventricle, septum, SA node, His bundle, right and left bundle branches, anterior and posterior hemibundles.

Right Coronary Artery (RCA)

Left Coronary Artery (LCA)

Left Circumflex Artery (Cx)

Left Anterior Descending (LAD)

1 mV/1 cm (standard calibration)

V6, MCL6   V3   AVF   III

V5   V2   AVL   II

V4   V1, MCL1   AVR   I

Myocardial Infarction ECG Patterns

(If signs of AMI are not present on the initial ECG
perform serial ECGs.)

Injury	Ischemia	Acute Infarction

(ST segments usually elevate within minutes of the onset of cardiac chest pain)	(T waves invert fully by 24 hours)	(Pathologic Q waves ≥.03 seconds or 1/3 height of QRS begin to form in 1 hour)

Old Infarction

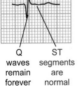

Q   ST
waves   segments
remain   are
forever   normal

Reciprocal ST Depression
(found in leads away from the infarction)

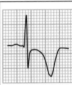

Non-Q-Wave Infarction
(flat, depressed ST segments in two or more contiguous leads; or may have inverted T waves)

NOTE: Early reperfusion is the definitive treatment for most AMI patients. The patient can lose 1% of salvageable myocardium for each minute of delay. Remember: "Time is Muscle."

Acute Anterior MI

(ST segment elevation ≥ 0.5–1 mm, with or without Q waves in two or more contiguous Leads: V_1–V_4. Poor R wave progression* and inverted T waves may also be present. Reciprocal ST depression may be present in: II, III, AVF.)

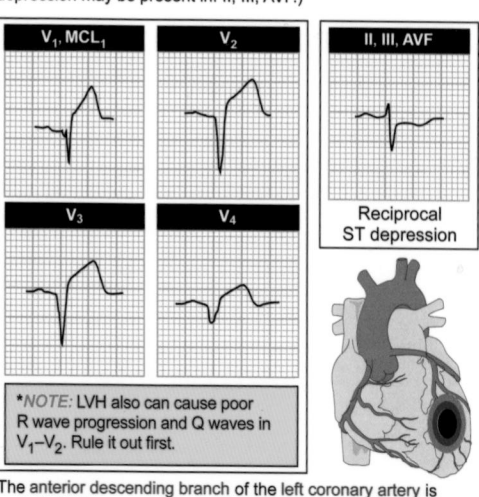

V_1, MCL_1	V_2	II, III, AVF
V_3	V_4	Reciprocal ST depression

*NOTE: LVH also can cause poor R wave progression and Q waves in V_1–V_2. Rule it out first.

The anterior descending branch of the left coronary artery is occluded. May cause: left anterior hemiblock; right bundle branch block; 2° AV block Mobitz II, 3° AV block with IVR, pump failure.

Third Degree Block

Acute Inferior MI

(ST segment elevation ≥0.5–1 mm in two or more contiguous Leads: II, III, AVF. Q waves and inverted T waves may also be present. Reciprocal ST depression may be present in Leads: I, AVL, V₂–V₄.)

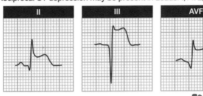

II	III	AVF

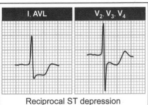

I, AVL	V₂, V₃, V₄

Reciprocal ST depression

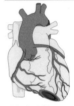

The right (or left) coronary artery is occluded. May cause: left posterior hemiblock; left axis deviation, ↓BP, sinus bradycardia, 1° AV block, 2° AV block Mobitz I (Wenckebach), **3° AV block with IJR.**

NOTE: Right ventricle AMI accompanies Inferior AMI 30% of the time. Check lead V₄R for elevated ST segment and Q wave.

3° block with IJR

Acute Right Ventricle MI

(ST segment elevation in Lead: V_4R (MCL_4R). Q wave and inverted T wave may also be present) Accompanies Inferior MI in 30% of cases.

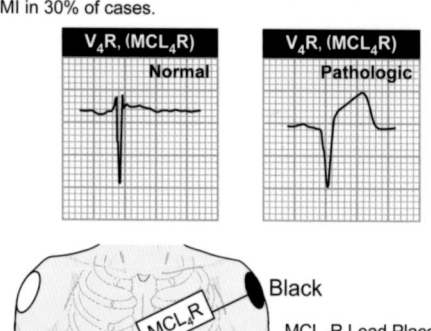

| V_4R, (MCL_4R) Normal | V_4R, (MCL_4R) Pathologic |

Black

MCL_4R

Red

MCL_4R Lead Placement: 5th interspace, right mid-clavicular line; monitor lead III.

RCA is occluded. May cause: AV block, A-Fib, A-Flutter, right heart failure, JVD with clear lungs, BP may drop if preload is reduced (be cautious with morphine, NTG, furosemide). Treat hypotension with IV fluids, pacing.

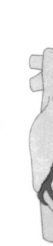

Acute Lateral MI

(ST segment elevation ≥0.5–1 mm in Leads: I, AVL, V_5, V_6. Q waves and inverted T waves may also be present)

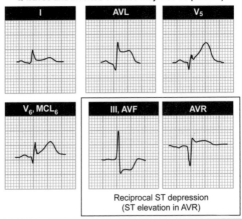

I	AVL	V_5

V_6, MCL_6	III, AVF	AVR

Reciprocal ST depression
(ST elevation in AVR)

NOTE: Lateral MI may be a component of a multiple site infarction, including anterior, inferior and/or posterior MI.

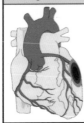

The circumflex branch of the left coronary artery is occluded. May cause: left ventricular dysfunction, AV nodal block.

Acute Posterior MI*

(ST segment depression with or without large R waves in Leads: V_1, V_2, V_3. Inverted T waves may also be present.)

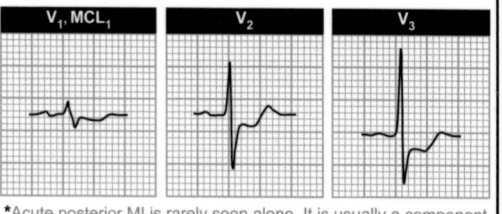

| V_1, MCL_1 | V_2 | V_3 |

*Acute posterior MI is rarely seen alone. It is usually a component of a multiple site infarction, including inferior MI. If suspected, obtain posterior chest leads V_7–V_9 for diagnoses.

NOTE: RVH can also cause a large R wave in V_1. Rule out RVH first.

The right coronary artery or the circumflex branch of the left coronary artery is occluded. May cause sinus arrest.

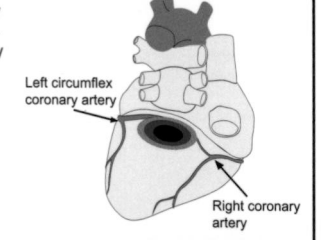

Left circumflex coronary artery

Right coronary artery

Sinus Arrest

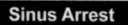

II

Bundle Branch Block

Left BBB
(Notched/slurred R waves in I, or V_5, or V_6. Qs in V_1)

I, V_5, V_6

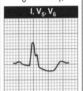

V_1, MCL_1

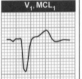

NOTE: If LBBB is present, do not attempt to diagnose AMI using only ECG criteria.

(QRS ≥ 0.12 second)

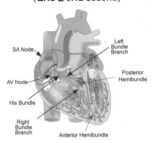

SA Node
AV Node
His Bundle
Right Bundle Branch
Left Bundle Branch
Posterior Hemibundle
Anterior Hemibundle

Right BBB
(Notched or two R waves in V_1 or V_2. Large S in I, V_5, V_6)

V_1, V_2, MCL_1 ### V_1, V_2, MCL_1

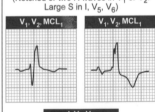

I, V_5, V_6

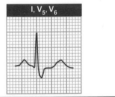

ACLS

Electrolyte/Drug Effects

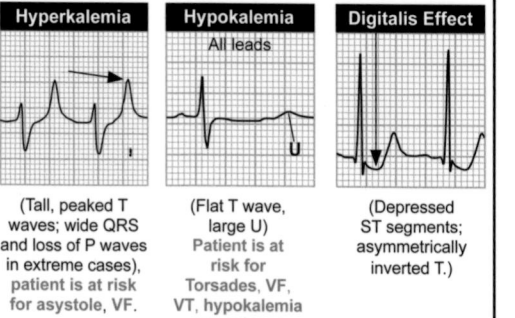

Hyperkalemia	Hypokalemia	Digitalis Effect
	All leads	

(Tall, peaked T waves; wide QRS and loss of P waves in extreme cases), patient is at risk for asystole, VF.

(Flat T wave, large U) Patient is at risk for Torsades, VF, VT, hypokalemia exacerbates digitalis toxicity.

(Depressed ST segments; asymmetrically inverted T.)

Torsades de Pointes

(2° anything that prolongs the QT interval: bradycardia, digitalis toxicity, quinidine, procainamide, disopyramide, phenothiazines, hypokalemia, hypomagnesemia, hypocalcemia, insecticide poisoning, subarachnoid hemorrhage, TCA OD.)

Medical Emergencies

Abbreviations Used In This Section

HX—History, Signs, and Symptoms
Key Symptoms and Findings (green text)
➕—Prehospital Treatment (blue text with yellow background)
❖—Medical Emergency
Intermediate Procedures (blue italicized text)
Cautions—Contraindications or Precautions (red text)

General History For Most Patients

Events that led up to the chief complaint? Past Hx?
Medications? Allergies? Known diseases? Dyspnea (SOB)?
Previous trauma or surgery? Nausea and Vomiting (N/V)?
Fever (Fv)? MedicAlert®?

Pain Questions

- ❑ Location, radiation?
- ❑ Speed and time of onset, duration?
- ❑ Nature, what type of pain, tenderness?
- ❑ What makes it better or worse?
- ❑ Any associated symptoms?
- ❑ Ever had this pain before? What was it? Rate pain on a 1–10 scale, 10 being worst.

General Treatment For Most Patients

- Follow your local protocols at all times.
- Ensure ABCs (Airway, Breathing, Circulation).
- Treat life- or limb-threatening injuries immediately.
- Get vital signs (pulse, BP, respirations, effort, lung sounds).
- Monitor O_2 saturation; give O_2 as needed; protect airway.
- *Perform Intermediate procedures, as indicated (IV, ECG, etc.).*
- Transport as soon as practical.
- Monitor patient's condition en route.
- Reassure and comfort your patient.

Abdominal Pain—Common Causes

- ❖ **Epigastric**: AMI, gastroenteritis, ulcer, esophageal disease, heartburn
- ❖ **LUQ**: gastritis, pancreatitis, AMI, pneumonia
- ❖ **LLQ**: ruptured ectopic pregnancy, ovarian cyst, PID, kidney stones, diverticulitis, enteritis, abdominal abscess
- ❖ **RLQ**: appendicitis, ruptured ectopic pregnancy, enteritis, diverticulitis, PID, ovarian cyst, kidney stones, abdominal abscess, strangulated hernia
- ❖ **RUQ**: gall stones, hepatitis, liver disease, pancreatitis, appendicitis, perforated duodenal ulcer, AMI, pneumonia
- ❖ **Midline**: bladder infection, aortic aneurysm, uterine disease, intestinal disease, early appendicitis
- ❖ **Diffuse Pain**: pancreatitis, peritonitis, appendicitis, gastroenteritis, dissecting/rupturing aortic aneurysm, diabetes, ischemic bowel, sickle cell crisis

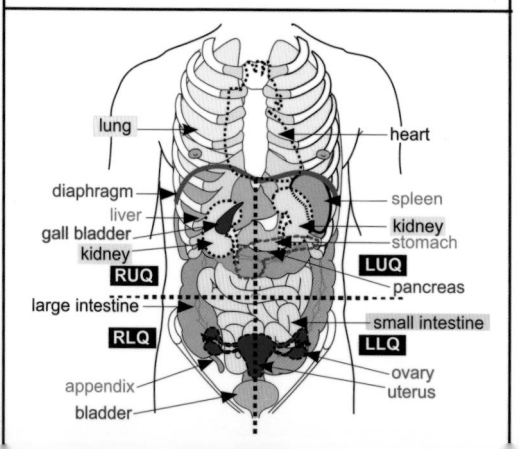

Abdominal Pain

HX—Ask Pain Questions and General History.
N/V? (color/quality of emesis)? Bowel movements, dysuria, menstrual Hx, fever, postural hypotension, referred shoulder pain? Is patient pregnant? Which trimester? Consider ectopic pregnancy. Genitourinary, vaginal, or rectal bleeding/discharge? Examine all 4 quadrants: abdominal tenderness, guarding, rigidity, bowel tones present? Distension, pulsatile mass? Record recent intake and GI habits. Vitals (sitting and supine), Chemstrip®. Peripheral pulses equal?

➕—Position of comfort and NPO. Consider pulse oximetry. O_2, IV (adjusted to vitals), consider ECG for epigastric pain.

CAUTION: Consider aortic aneurysm; ectopic pregnancy, DKA. Epigastric abdominal pain may be cardiac.

- ❖ **Abdominal Aortic Aneurysm**: Severe abdominal pain, pulsatile mass, hypotension.
- ❖ **Acute MI**: Chest "pressure" or epigastric pain radiating to left arm or jaw, diaphoresis, N/V, SOB, pallor, dysrhythmias.
- ❖ **Appendicitis**: N/V, RLQ or periumbilical pain, fever, shock.
- ❖ **Bowel Obstruction**: N/V (fecal odor), localized pain.
- ❖ **Cholecystitis**: Acute onset RUQ pain and tenderness (may be referred to right shoulder/scapula)—may be related to high-fat meal. N/V, anorexia, fever. "Female, fat, 40."
- ❖ **Ectopic Pregnancy**: Missed period, pelvic pain, abnormal vaginal bleeding, dizziness.
- ❖ **Food Poisoning**: N/V, diffuse abdominal pain and cramping, diarrhea, fever, weakness, dizziness. Severe symptoms: descending paralysis, respiratory compromise.
- ❖ **Hepatic Failure**: Jaundice, confusion/coma, edema, bleeding and bruising, renal failure, fever, anorexia, dehydration.

Medical

- ❖ **Kidney Stone**: Constant or colicky severe flank pain, extreme restlessness, hematuria, N/V.
- ❖ **Pancreatitis**: Severe, "sharp," or "twisting" epigastric or LUQ pain radiating to back. N/V, diaphoresis, abdominal distention, signs of shock, fever.
- ❖ **Ulcer**: "Burning," epigastric pain, N/V, possible hematemesis, hypotension, decreased bowel sounds.

Notes

Abuse

✚—Remove the patient from the environment, transport to hospital. Report possible abuse to police, ED staff, protective services, and appropriate authorities. Call for police assistance, if needed, to protect the patient, and remove him/her from the scene. Do not confront the alleged abuser. Document your findings and any statements made by patient, family members, and others. Provide medical care, as needed. If sexual abuse is suspected, do not allow the patient to wash.

Non-Accidental Child Maltreatment

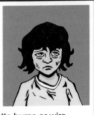

HX—Any unusual MOI, or one that does not match the child's injury/illness. Parents may accuse the child of hurting himself/herself, or may be vague/contradictory in providing history. There may be a delay in seeking medical care. The child may not cling to mother. Fracture in any child <2 years old; multiple injuries in various stages of healing, or on many parts of the body; obvious cigarette burns or wire marks; malnutrition; insect infestation, chronic skin infection, unkempt child. Head injury is the leading cause of death of abused children.

Intimate Partner Violence

HX—Repeated ED visits with injuries becoming more severe with each visit. Minimizing the seriousness or frequency of the injuries. Seeking treatment one or more days after the injuries. Injuries that are not likely to have been caused by the accident reported. Overprotective significant other who does not allow the patient to be alone with the health care professional. Fractures in different stages of healing, according to radiographic findings. History of child abuse to patient or partner.

Older Adult Maltreatment

HX—Fractures or bruises at various stages of healing. Unexplained bruises or cigarette burns on the torso or extremities. Soft tissue injuries from signs of restraint use. Head injuries. Malnourishment, listlessness, unexplained dehydration. Poor hygiene, inappropriate clothing. Decubitus ulcer, urine and feces on body and clothing. Unusual interaction between caregiver and patient.

✚—Remove the patient from the environment. Transport to hospital. Report possible abuse to police, ED staff, protective services, and appropriate authorities. Call for police assistance, if needed, to protect the patient and remove him/her from the scene. Do not confront the alleged abuser. Document your findings and any statements made by patient, family members, others. Provide medical care, as needed. If sexual abuse is suspected, do not allow the patient to wash.

Airway Obstruction

See "CHOKING."

Allergic Reaction

HX—Mild reaction (local swelling only) or serious systemic reaction (hives, pallor, bronchospasm, wheezing, upper airway obstruction with stridor, swelling of throat, hypotension). If cardiac arrest, treat per ACLS.

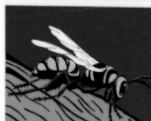

✚—If bee sting, remove stinger.
* For mild local reaction: wash area, apply cold pack.
* For serious reaction: secure airway, ventilate, O_2; large bore IV, titrate to BP >90; ECG; **Epinephrine: Adult epinephrine: 1:1,000 0.3-0.5 mg IM; Pediatric: 0.01 mg/kg IM [0.3 mL maximum]).** Consider IV diphenhydramine and steroids for severe reactions.

Cautions—Epinephrine may cause arrhythmias or angina.

Altered Mental Status

Consider: Hypoglycemia, CVA/TIA, postictal, alcohol, drugs, hypovolemia, head injury, hypothermia, HazMat, sepsis, shock, cardiogenic, vasovagal.

HX—Ask **Pain Questions and General History**. Time of onset: slow or fast? Seizure activity? Was patient sitting, standing, lying? Is patient pregnant (consider ectopic pregnancy)? Any recent illness or trauma? Current level of consciousness? Neurological status and psychological status? Any vomiting (bloody or coffee-ground)? Melena (black tarry stool)? Any signs of recent trauma?

⊞—**General treatment**: Protect airway. Give O_2 as needed. Be prepared to assist ventilations. GCS <8? Intubate. Monitor ECG, vitals.

⊞—**Cardiac: Support ABCs**. Vitals, O_2, treat per ACLS.

⊞—**Coma:** (If multiple patients, suspect toxins—protect yourself!) Any odor at scene?—Consider HazMat. Were there any preceding symptoms or H/A? Past Hx: HTN, diabetes? Medications? Check scene for pill bottles or syringes and bring along. Get vitals, LOC and neuro findings, pupils. Any signs of trauma, drug abuse? Skin: color, temperature, rash, welts, facial or extremity asymmetry? MedicAlert® tag?

WARNING: Ensure your safety first, then the safety of patient and others.

- Secure airway, ventilate with 100% O_2, protect C-spine
- Start IV. Get Chemstrip®. Consider glucose, naloxone
- Monitor vital signs, O_2 saturation, and ECG

Cautions—Protect airway, suction as needed.

⊞—**Sepsis/Infection**: O_2, IV, vitals. IV fluids for hypotension.

⊞—**Syncope**: Position of comfort, O_2, IV, vitals, ECG. Consider IV fluids for hypotension.

Cautions—Syncope in middle-aged or elderly patients is often cardiac. Occult internal bleeding may cause syncope.

Childbirth (See also, OB/GYN Emergencies)

HX—Timing of contractions? Intensity? Does mother have urge to push or to move bowels? Has amniotic sac ruptured? Medications—any medical problems? Vital signs—check for:

- Vaginal bleeding or amniotic fluid; note color of fluid
- Crowning (means imminent delivery)
- Abnormal presentation (foot, arm, breech, cord, shoulder)

NOTE: Transport immediately if patient has had previous C-section, known multiple births, any abnormal presentation, excessive bleeding, or if pregnancy is not full-term and child will be premature.

➕—**Normal:** Control delivery using gloved hand to guide head, suction mouth and nose, deliver, keep infant level with perineum, clamp and cut cord 8"–10" from infant, **warm and dry infant**, stimulate infant by drying with towel, **make sure respirations are adequate.** Normal VS are: pulse: >120, respirations: >40, BP: 70, weight: 3.5 kg. Give baby

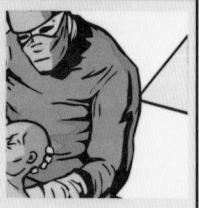

to mother to nurse at breast. Get APGAR scores at 1 and 5 minutes after birth. If excessive post-partum bleeding, treat for shock, massage uterus to aid contraction, have mother nurse infant, **start large bore IV**, consider oxytocin 10–40 units in 1,000 mL NS IV. Transport without waiting for placenta to deliver. Bring it with you to the hospital. Obtain mother's vital signs, O_2 saturation.

NOTE: Most births are normal—reassure mom and dad.

➕—**Breech:** Call OLMC. If head will not deliver, consider applying gentle pressure on mother's abdomen. Support legs and buttocks of baby; during contraction pull gently on baby. Encourage mother to pant, not push. If unsuccessful, insert your gloved fingers in vagina; deliver one shoulder, then the other. Do not pull on baby at this stage.

Deliver head by supporting baby's chest with your arms and hands. Place your fingers in vagina and find baby's mouth. Grasp the chin and apply gentle upward pressure to head and shoulders. Apply suprapubic pressure as well. If baby will not deliver, place fingers between baby's face and vaginal wall to create airway. Rapid transport—patient may need emergency C-section.

+—Cord Presents: Call OLMC. Place mother in trendelenburg or knee-chest position, hold pressure on baby's head to relieve pressure on cord, check pulses in cord, keep cord moist with saline dressing, O_2, rapid transport, **start IV en route**. Patient may require emergency C-section.

+—Foot/Leg Presents: Call OLMC. Support presenting part, place mother in trendelenburg or knee-chest position, O_2, **start IV**. Rapid transport.

+—Cord Around Neck: Unwrap cord from neck and deliver normally, keep face clear, suction mouth and nose, etc.

+—Infant Not Breathing: Stimulate with dry towel, rub back, flick soles of feet with finger. **Suction mouth and nose. Ventilate with BVM and 100% O_2** (this will revive most infants). Begin chest compressions if HR <60. If child does not respond, contact OLMC and reassess quality of ventilation efforts, lung sounds (pneumothorax? obstruction?) O_2 connected? **Intubate and ventilate.** Epinephrine 0.01 mg/kg IV/IO, or 0.1 mg/kg 1:1,000 ET; and IV fluids 10 mL/kg, glucose 2 mL/kg D25%W. Rapid transport. See *Peds section, Pediatric Arrest*.

Cautions—Failure to respond usually indicates hypoxia—**airway management is paramount in neonates**.

APGAR Scale

	0 points	1 point	2 points	1 Min	5 Min
Heart rate	Absent	<100	>100		
Resp. Effort	Absent	Slow, Irregular	Strong cry		
Muscle Tone	Flaccid	Some flex	Active motion		
Irritability	No response	Some	Vigorous		
Color	Blue, pale	Body: pink Extremities: Blue	Fully pink		
			TOTAL:		

Infants with scores of 7–10 usually require supportive care only. **A score of 4–6 indicates moderate depression.**

NOTE: Infants with scores of 3 or less require aggressive resuscitation.

Notes

OB/GYN Emergencies

❖ **Abruptio Placenta**: Separation of placenta from uterine wall. Usually occurs >20 weeks gestation. Painful 3rd trimester vaginal bleeding (dark red), hypovolemic shock, hypotension, tachycardia, fetal distress. ↓FHT, ↑fundal height, pale skin, diaphoresis.

➕ —IV, O_2, rapid transport—patient may require emergency C-section.

❖ **Placenta Previa**: Placenta covers cervical os, can occur during 2nd and 3rd trimester. Painless bright red vaginal bleeding, possible hypotension, tachycardia.

➕ —O_2, IV, OB consult; if bleeding is heavy, rapid transport—patient may require C-section.

❖ **Preeclampsia/PIH**: (Pregnancy induced hypertension). HTN, H/A, proteinuria, edema of hands, feet, face and sacrum, weight gain, ↓urine output, visual disturbances, possible ↑liver enzymes, ↑neurologic reflexes, ↑chance of seizures, ↓FHT.

➕ —Transport quietly and gently, vitals, IV; treat HTN with labetalol, seizure prophylaxis with magnesium sulfate; OB consult, supportive care.

Physiologic Changes of Pregnancy

BP	Pulse	CO	ECG	Respirations	ABG	Blood Work	Other
↓	↑	↑	T Wave changes L II, avF, avL	↑Resp Rate ↑Tidal Volume ↓Vital Capacity ↓Functional residual capacity	↑pH ↑PaO2 ↓PaCO2 ↓HCO3 Respiratory Alkalosis	↓HCT, ↑WBC ↑Fibrinogen ↑Clotting factors, Prone to DIC, ↑Blood Volume	↑N/V, aspiration ↑Injury: uterus, pelvis, bladder ↑Falls ↑Peripheral venous pressure

54

Maternal Cardiac Arrest

Activate Maternal Cardiac Arrest Team (document start time)
Consider and Treat Causes❖ (below)
Assess C-A-B, secure airway, give 100% O₂

⇩

Start CPR (hand placement higher on sternum than usual.
Defibrillate as usual—See *ACLS section, Adult Cardiac Arrest*
Give standard ACLS drugs and doses
If receiving IV/IO magnesium, stop infusion and give
1 gm calcium chloride 10% (10 mL) IV/IO *OR:*
3 gm calcium gluconate 10% (30 mL) IV/IO.
Start IV above the diaphragm—fluid bolus for hypovolemia

Experienced provider for advanced airway placement:
• may require smaller ET tube
• monitor for airway bleeding
• preoxygenate to prevent hypoxia
• RSI preferred
• choose sedative that will minimize hypotension

Monitor waveform capnography and CPR.
If PETCO₂ <10, improve CPR.
If obvious gravid uterus: ⇨
• Manually displace uterus to left to relieve
  aortocaval compression
• Remove any internal and external fetal
  monitors
• Prepare for emergency cesarean
  section if no ROSC in 4 minutes

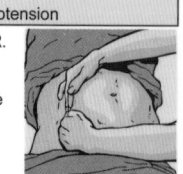

manual left uterine
displacement

• **Goal: delivery within 5 minutes of
  beginning CPR**
• Continue maternal resuscitation during and after C-section

❖ Special Causes:

• Acidosis	• HTN/Eclampsia	• Placenta Abruption
• Amniotic fluid embolus	• Hyper/Hypokalemia	• Placenta Previa
• Anesthetic effects	• Hypothermia	• Sepsis
• Bleeding	• Hypovolemia	• Tension Pneumothorax
• Cardiac disease	• Hypoxia	• Toxins
• Cardiac tamponade	• MI	• Uterine Atony
• DIC	• PE	

Vaginal Bleeding (See also, OB/GYN Emergencies)

❖—Consider: **Miscarriage**, **ectopic pregnancy**, also **CA**, **trauma**.

HX—Ask **Pain Questions and General History**. Cramping? Clots, tissue fragments (bring to ER), dizziness, weakness, thirst (painless bleeding with pregnancy suggests placenta previa). Duration, amount; last menstrual period (normal or irregular)? If patient is pregnant: due date? **Past HX**— Bleeding problems, pregnancies, medications? Vitals and orthostatic change? Fever? Evidence of blood loss, signs of shock? Vasoconstriction, sweating, altered mental status.

✚—**General Treatment**: O_2, IV large bore, titrated to vitals, assess vitals, O_2 saturation, ECG.

Cautions—If miscarriage is suspected, field vaginal exam is generally not indicated.

✚—**Postpartum Bleeding**: Treat for shock, massage uterus to aid contraction, have mother nurse infant, start large bore IV, transport without waiting for placenta to deliver. Bring it with you to the hospital. Get vital signs.

✚—**Abruptio Placenta**: Painful 3rd trimester bleeding. Look for hypovolemic shock, give O_2, start IV. Rapid transport.

✚—**Placenta Previa**: Painless 3rd trimester bleeding. Start IV, O_2. Rapid transport.

Medical

Chest Pain

❖—**Consider: AMI, CHF, APE, pneumothorax, pneumonia, bronchitis, pulmonary embolus**. **HX**—Ask **Pain Questions and General History**. Syncope, dizziness, weakness, diaphoresis? Fever, pallor? Dyspnea? **Past Hx**: Chest trauma? Cardiac or respiratory problems, diabetes, high blood pressure, heart failure? Lung sounds, JVD? Peripheral or pulmonary edema? General appearance?

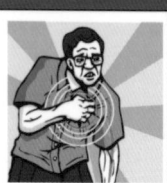

➕ —Position of comfort, reassure patient, vitals, O_2 PRN, ECG, IV. Consider nitroglycerine for cardiac chest pain: 0.4 mg SL every 5 minutes (maximum: 3 doses). Consider aspirin for AMI.

IMPORTANT: Notify ED if your cardiac patient is a possible fibrinolytic candidate, and transport ASAP.

Cautions—Treat dysrhythmias according to ACLS.

❖ **Acute MI**: Severe, crushing chest pain, or substernal "pressure," radiating to the left arm, or jaw. N/V, SOB, diaphoresis, pallor, dysrhythmias, HTN or hypotension.
❖ **Aortic Dissection**: Sudden onset "tearing" chest or back pain, tachycardia, HTN or hypotension, possible unequal pulses or unequal BP in extremities.
❖ **Cholecystitis**: Acute onset RUQ pain and tenderness (may be referred to right shoulder/scapula)—may be elated to high-fat meal; N/V, anorexia, fever. "Female, fat, 40."
❖ **Hiatal Hernia**: Positional epigastric pain.
❖ **Musculo-Skeletal**: Pain on palpation, respiration. Obvious signs of trauma.
❖ **Pleurisy**: Pain on inspiration, fever, pleural friction rub.
❖ **Pneumonia**: Fever, shaking, chills, pleuritic chest pain, crackles, productive cough, tachycardia, diaphoresis.
❖ **Pulmonary Embolus**: Sudden onset SOB, cough, chest pain which is sharp and pleuritic, tachycardia, rapid respirations, O_2 sat <94%, apprehension, diaphoresis, hemoptysis, crackles.
❖ **Ulcer**: "Burning" epigastric pain, N/V, possible hematemesis, hypotension, decreased bowel sounds.

Notes

CPR—Adult, Child, or Infant

1. **Unresponsive?** (not breathing, or only gasping?)
2. **Call for assistance**—have someone get defibrillator/AED
3. **Check pulse within 10 seconds** (if present, give 1 breath every 5–6 seconds; check pulse every 2 minutes)— *if NO PULSE:*
4. **Position patient supine** on hard, flat surface
5. **Begin chest compression**s, 30:2, push hard and fast 100–120/min., allow full chest recoil—minimize interruptions
6. **Open airway:** head-tilt/chin-lift, ventilate x2* (avoid excessive ventilations)
7. **Attach AED** to adult (and child >1 year old)

Shockable rhythm?

Yes ← → **No**

Yes	No
8. **Shock x1**	8. **Resume CPR immediately** x2 minutes
9. **Resume CPR immediately** x2 minutes	9. **Initiate ALS interventions**
10. **Check rhythm**— *if shockable:*	10. **Check rhythm** every 2 minutes
11. **Shock x1;** resume CPR	

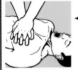

lower half of sternum

head-tilt/chin-lift

CPR	Ratio	Rate	Depth	Check Pulse
Adult: 1 Person	30:2	100–120	2–2.4"	Carotid
Adult: 2 Person	30:2	100–120	2–2.4"	Carotid
Child: 1 Person	30:2	100–120	1/3 cx or 2"	Carotid
Child: 2 Person	15:2	100–120	1/3 cx or 2"	Carotid
Infant: 1 Person	30:2	100–120	1/3 cx or 1.5"	Brachial, Fem.
Infant: 2 Person	15:2	100–120	1/3 cx or 1.5"	Brachial, Fem.
Newborn: 2 Person	3:1	100–120	1/3 cx or 1.5"	Brachial, Fem.

*Adult—once an advanced airway is placed, ventilate at 8–10/minute.

Medical

Choking

For Responsive Choking Adult Or Child >1 Year

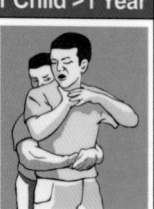

1. If patient cannot talk or has stridor, or cyanosis
2. **Perform Heimlich Maneuver** (use chest thrusts if patient is pregnant or obese), repeat until successful or patient is unconscious
3. **Begin CPR/call for assistance**
4. **Open airway; head-tilt/chin-lift** (look and remove object, if visible)
5. **Ventilate with two breaths,** if unable
6. **Reposition head; attempt to ventilate,** if unable
7. **Perform chest compressions (30:2)**
8. **Repeat: inspect mouth → remove object → ventilate → chest compressions** until successful
9. **Consider** laryngoscopy and removal of object by forceps, ET intubation, transtracheal ventilation, cricothyrotomy
10. If patient resumes breathing, place in the recovery position

For Unresponsive Choking Adult Or Child

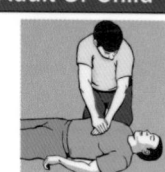

1. **Determine unresponsiveness**
2. **Call for assistance**
3. **Position patient supine** on hard, flat surface
4. **Open airway**—head-tilt/chin-lift (look and remove object if visible)
5. **Attempt to ventilate,** if unable
6. **Reposition head and chin, attempt to ventilate,** if unable
7. **Begin chest compressions (30:2)**
8. **Repeat: inspect mouth → remove object → ventilate → chest compressions** until successful
9. **Consider** laryngoscopy and removal of object by forceps, ET intubation, transtracheal ventilation, cricothyrotomy
10. If patient resumes breathing, place in the recovery position

For Choking Infant

1. **Confirm obstruction**: if infant can not make sounds, breathe, cry or is cyanotic
2. **Invert infant on arm**: support head by cupping face in hand; **perform 5 back slaps and 5 chest thrusts** until object is expelled
3. **Repeat until successful**
4. **If patient becomes unconscious, start CPR**
5. **Open airway, and ventilate x2**—if unable
6. **Reposition head and chin, attempt to ventilate again**
7. **Begin chest compressions (30:2)**
8. **Consider** laryngoscopy and removal of object by forceps, ET intubation, transtracheal ventilation, cricothyrotomy
9. **If patient resumes breathing, place in the recovery position**

Drowning and Near Drowning

HX—How long was patient submerged? Fresh or salt water? Cold water (<40°F)? Diving accident? Immobilize spine. Vitals, pulse oximetry, neurological status, GCS, crackles or pulmonary edema with respiratory distress?

⊕—Open airway, suction, assist ventilations, start CPR. C-Spine: stabilize before removing patient from water. O_2, IV, monitor ECG. If hypothermic: use heated O_2 and follow hypothermia protocols. Conserve heat with blankets.

Cautions—All unconscious patients should have **C-spine immobilization**. All near-drowning patients should be transported. Many deteriorate later and develop pulmonary edema.

NOTE: Prepare for vomiting; intubate if unconscious.

Medical

Hyperglycemia

HX—Slow onset, excessive urination, thirst; When was insulin last taken? Abdominal cramps, N/V, mental status, high glucose on Chemstrip®, skin signs, dehydration? Respirations: deep and rapid? Breath odor: acetone, fruity?

⊕—Secure airway, vital signs, O₂, large bore IV, fluid challenge (balanced salt solution). Monitor ECG.

Hypoglycemia/Insulin Shock

HX—Sudden onset, low blood glucose on Chemstrip®. Last insulin dose? Last meal? Mental status? Diaphoresis, H/A, blurred vision, dizziness, tachycardia, tremors, seizures?

⊕—Support ABCs, O₂, PRN, vitals, IV. Give 50mL D50W% if patient is comatose (perform Chemstrip® before and after). Consider glucagon 1 mg IM if unable to start IV. **Do not give oral glucose if airway is compromised.**

Cautions—Hypoglycemia can mimic a stroke or intoxication. Seizures, coma, and confusion are common symptoms. When in doubt about the diagnosis, give glucose IV or PO.

	HYPOGLYCEMIA	HYPERGLYCEMIA
Also known as	"Insulin Shock"	"Ketoacidosis," "DKA"
Incidence	More common	Less common
Blood sugar	Low (≤ 80 mg%)	High (≥180 mg%)
Onset	Rapid (minutes)	Gradual (days)
Skin	Moist, pale	Dry, warm
Respirations	Normal	Deep or rapid
Pulse	Normal or fast	Rapid, weak
Blood Pressure	Normal or high	Normal or low
Breath odor	Normal	Ketone/Acetone odor
Seizures	Common	Uncommon
Dehydration	No	Yes
Urine Output	Normal	Excessive
Thirst	Normal	Very Thirsty
Mental Status	Disoriented, Coma	Awake, weak, tired
Treatment	Glucose IV or PO	IV Fluids, Insulin, K⁺
Recovery	Rapid (minutes)	Gradual (days)

Hyperthermia/Heat Stroke

HX—Onset? Exercise or drug (cocaine) induced? Vitals, temperature, skin: warm, dry?

➕—Remove from hot environment. Evaluate airway. Undress and begin cooling patient. Consider cold packs to groin, armpits. **Evaporation and convection measures work best** (but avoid causing shivering, as this may increase patient temperature). Start large bore IV. Consider fluid challenge. Monitor ECG. Reassess vital signs en route.

Cautions—Rapid cooling is key. Consider ice bath submersion.

Hypothermia (See also, ACLS section, Hypothermia)

HX—Vital signs, mental status. Is patient cold? Shivering? Evidence of local injury?
Mild hypothermia: Shivering, ↑HR, ↑RR, lethargy, confusion.
Moderate hypothermia: ↓Respirations, ↓HR, rigidity, LOC, "J wave" on ECG.
Severe hypothermia: Coma, ↓BP, ↓HR, acidosis, VF, systole.

➕—Secure airway. Remove patient from cold environment **Give heated O$_2$**. A severely hypothermic patient may breathe slowly. Monitor ECG, large bore IV. **If cardiac arrest, start CPR** (see also, *ACLS section, Hypothermia*). Contact OLMC. Cut wet clothing off (do not pull off), wrap patient with blankets. Record vital signs, including temperature.

Cautions—Handle patient gently. Jostling can cause cardiac arrest. **If patient is not shivering, do not ambulate**. Stimulating the airway can cause cardiac arrest.

Medical

Infectious Diseases

Disease	Spread By	Risk To You
AIDS/HIV	IV/Sex/Blood products	↓Immune function, Pneumonias, Cancer
Anthrax	*Cutaneous:* contact with skin lesions	Infection = 25% mortality, but much lower if treated
	Ingestion: eating contaminated meat	Infection = high mortality, unless treated with antibiotics
	Pulmonary: inhaled spores	Infection = 95% mortality, but much lower if treated
C-diff	Secretions/Excretions Hand to nose	Diarrhea, nausea, shock
Hepatitis A*	Fecal-oral	Acute hepatitis, jaundice
Hepatitis B*	IV/Sex/Birth/Blood	Acute and chronic hepatitis, cirrhosis, liver CA
Hepatitis C	Blood	Chronic hepatitis, cirrhosis, liver CA
Hepatitis D	IV/Sex/Birth	Chronic liver disease
Hepatitis E	Fecal-oral	↑Mortality to pregnant women and fetus
Herpes	Skin contact	Skin lesions, shingles
Influenza	Droplet/Airborne	Fever, pneumonia, prostration
MRSA	Secretions/ Excretions Hand to nose	Ulceration, tissue destruction
Meningitis*	Nasal secretions	Low risk to rescuer
Norovirus	Fecal to oral Hand to mouth	Diarrhea, nausea, vomiting
Tuberculosis	Sputum/cough/ Airborne	Cough, weight loss, lung damage
Zika virus	Mosquito bites	Fever, rash, joint pain, red eyes, muscle pain, headache, infection during pregnancy can cause certain birth defects

- Wear gloves for all patient contacts and for all contacts with body fluids.
- Wash hands after patient contact.
- Place a mask on patients who are coughing or sneezing.
- Place a mask on yourself.
- Wear eye shields or goggles when body fluids may splash.
- Wear gowns when needed.
- Wear utility gloves for cleaning equipment.
- Do not recap, cut, or bend needles.

CAUTION: Report every exposure and get immediate treatment!

Notes

Organ and Tissue Donation

TISSUE	AGE	RESTRICTIONS
Bone	15–75	No IV drug use, no malignancy, no transmissible disease
Eyes	Any age	No systemic infection, no IV drug use, no transmissible disease
Heart valves	NB–55	No IV drug use, no transmissible disease
Organs	NB–70	Brain dead or potential to meet brain death, ventilator-dependent
Skin	15–75	No IV drug use, no malignancy, no transmissible disease

NOTE: There are very few contraindications to donation.

Psychiatric Emergencies

HX—Recent crisis? Emotional trauma, suicidal, changes in behavior, drug/alcohol abuse? Toxins, head injury, diabetes, seizure disorder, sepsis or other illness? Ask about suicidal feelings, intent; does patient have a plan? Make judgement about whether patient will act on plan. Vitals, pupil signs, mental status, oriented? Any odor on breath? MedicAlert®? Any signs of trauma?

IMPORTANT: Make sure scene is safe—protect yourself!

✚—Contact OLMC or psychiatric hospital. ABCs. Restrain patient as needed. If patient is suicidal, do not leave alone. Remove dangerous objects (weapons, pills, etc.). Transport in calm, quiet manner, if possible. Consider: O₂, IV, check blood sugar. If low, consider glucose PO or IV.

CAUTION: Always suspect hypoglycemia, and look for other medical causes: ETOH, drugs, sepsis, CVA, etc.

Respiratory Distress

HX—Ask Pain Questions and General History. Onset of event: was it slow or fast? Fever? Cough? Is cough productive? Recent respiratory infection? Does patient smoke (how much)? Record patient's medications. Assess severity of dyspnea (mild, moderate, severe) and tidal volume. Single word sentences? Is cyanosis present? Level of consciousness? Lung sounds: any wheezing, crackles, rhonchi, diminished sounds? Vitals? Pulse oximetry. Is patient exhausted? Candidate for intubation? Upper airway obstruction (stridor, hoarseness, drooling, coughing)? Chest pain? Itching, hives? Numbness of mouth and hands? Signs of CHF: JVD, wet lung sounds (crackles), peripheral edema?

➕—**General treatment**: Position of comfort (usually upright). Give O_2 as needed. Be prepared to assist ventilations. Monitor ECG, vitals. Start IV, SaO_2, End-Tidal CO_2.

Cautions—High flow O_2 can depress respirations in a patient with COPD. Prepare to assist respirations.

❖ **Anaphylaxis**: See **ALLERGIC REACTION**

❖ **Asthma**: "Wheezes"

➕—Consider nebulized bronchodilators, and/or epinephrine 1:1,000 SQ (0.3 mg–0.5 mg). Consider Atrovent, steroids.

❖ **COPD**: "Wheezes, rhonchi."

➕—Consider nebulized bronchodilators. Consider Atrovent, steroids.

❖ **Pulmonary Edema**:

➕—Consider nebulized bronchodilators, furosemide, sublingual nitroglycerine, morphine, and CPAP.

❖ **Tension Pneumothorax**:

➕—Contact OLMC. Lift occlusive dressing, needle thoracentesis. Rapid transport.

Scene Safety

CAUTION: Wait until police secure the scene before entering: intimate partner violence, assault, any shooting or stabbing.

❑ As you approach, scan the area for hazards such as: hostile persons, dogs, uncontrolled traffic, spilled chemicals, gas, oil, down power lines
❑ Keep your exit routes open
❑ Any weapons present at the scene should be secured
❑ Wear protective gear. Call for more resources if needed

Crime Scene

IMPORTANT: Consider the safety of your crew first. Consider staging out of sight until scene is secure.

Access and Treatment

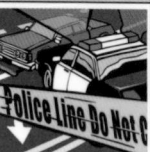

1. Consult with police regarding best access.
2. Make a mental note of physical and weather conditions.
3. Do not park your vehicle over visible tire tracks.
4. To avoid destroying evidence, select a single route to and from the victim.
5. Limit the number of personnel allowed on scene.
6. Be conscious of any statements made.
7. Do not cut through any holes in patients' clothing.
8. Place victim on a clean sheet for transport. After transport, obtain the sheet, fold it onto itself, and give to the police.
9. When moving the victim, it is important to note:
   • Location of furniture prior to moving
   • Position of victim prior to moving
   • Status of clothing
   • Location of any weapons or other articles
   • Name of personnel who moved items
10. Consult with police regarding whether to pick up medical debris left over from treatment.
11. Write a detailed report regarding your crews actions.

Seizures

❖ Consider **epilepsy**, hypoxia, **CVA**, **cardiac origin**, **ETOH/drug use/withdrawal**, **hypoglycemia**, **pregnancy**, **hyperthermia**, **infection**, or **metabolic cause**.

HX—Type (generalized or partial), onset, length, seizure history or meds? Compliance? Recent head trauma? What was patient doing before seizure? Did patient fall? Bite tongue? Dysrhythmias? Incontinent? Is seizure drug-induced (antidepressant cocaine)? MedicAlert®? Level of consciousness? Head or oral trauma? Focal neurologic signs? H/A? Respiratory status?

✛— **Generalized**: Keep airway open, consider NPA (do not use EOA/EGTA), O₂, suction, IV, test CBG, consider IV glucose, benzodiazepines as needed, transport on side. Monitor ECG, vitals.

✛—**Partial**: Do not grab patient; may lead to violent reaction. Block patient's access to doors, windows, etc. Direct, do not restrain. Use calm reassurance. Establish LOC. Monitor recovery.

✛—**Patient having seizure who has VNS implant**: Pass patient's wrist magnet over VNS (Vagus Nerve Stimulator) on slow 3-second count. Implant usually in upper left chest. Repeat every 3–5 minutes, maximum of 3 times. If VNS does not stop seizure, treat per **Generalized** guidelines above.

Cautions—Seizure in water can lead to APE. Transport for evaluation. Restrain patient only to prevent injury—protect patient's head. Do not force anything into the mouth. Always check for a pulse after seizure stops. Most seizures are self-limiting, lasting less than 1–2 minutes.

NOTE: Not all patients having a seizure need transport.

Shock

HX—Ask **Pain Questions and General History**. Onset?
Associated symptoms: hives, edema, thirst, weakness,
dyspnea, chest pain, dizziness when upright, abdominal pain?
Trauma? Bloody vomitus or stools? Delayed capillary refill?
Tachypnea? Syncope? N/V? Mental status: confusion,
restlessness? Tachycardia, hypotension? Skin: pale,
sweaty, cool. Signs of pump failure: JVD while upright,
crackles, peripheral edema.

✚—Stop hemorrhage, if any. Apply direct pressure to
wound. Consider pressure point or tourniquet. Place patient
supine, O_2 PRN, assist ventilations as needed, Start large
bore IV. Do not delay transport to start IV. (Consider
intraosseous infusion if unable to start IV.) Prevent heat
loss. Try to determine the type of shock (hypovolemic,
cardiogenic, obstructive, distributive, etc.). **If trauma, enter
patient in Trauma System**. Assess lung sounds. Monitor
ECG, O_2 sat, vitals, level of consciousness.

Cautions—Check lung sounds for crackles before giving IV
fluids and after each bolus.

Notes

Stroke/CVA

HX—New neuro symptoms <24 hours? Ambulatory at baseline? Preceding symptoms: headache, confusion, seizure, dizziness, loss of balance or coordination, trouble walking, sudden onset of numbness or weakness of the face, arm, or leg (especially on one side of the body), trouble speaking or seeing in one or both eyes? **Past HX**— HTN, Diabetes, seizure? **Findings**: Age >45 years, LOC, GCS, patient aware of name? MedicAlert® tag? CBG >60 and <400, pupils, vitals, meds? Neuro: Facial droop-smile/ grimice, slurred speech, difficulty understanding, hand grips, arm or leg drift, weakness, or paralysis?

⊕—Airway, O₂ PRN, suction and assist ventilations as needed. IV, GCS, check blood glucose and give IV glucose, if hypoglycemic. Vitals, ECG (CVA may be 2° to cardiac event).

Patient may be candidate for fibrinolysis. Consider rapid transport. Complete LAPSS.

Brain Areas

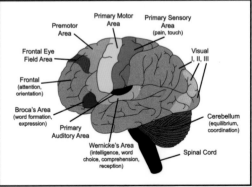

Premotor Area

Primary Motor Area

Primary Sensory Area (pain, touch)

Frontal Eye Field Area

Visual I, II, III

Frontal (attention, orientation)

Broca's Area (word formation, expression)

Primary Auditory Area

Cerebellum (equilibrium, coordination)

Wernicke's Area (intelligence, word choice, comprehension, reception)

Spinal Cord

Medical

Posturing

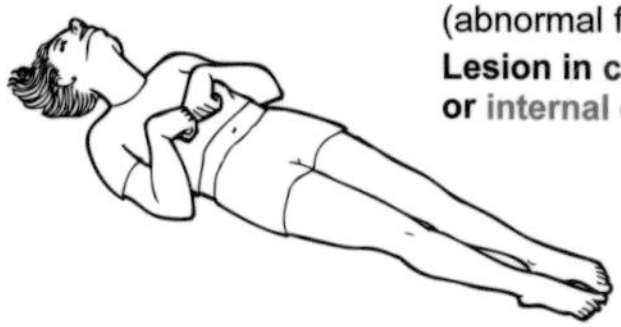

Decorticate:
(abnormal flexion)
**Lesion in cerebral hemispheres
or** internal capsule

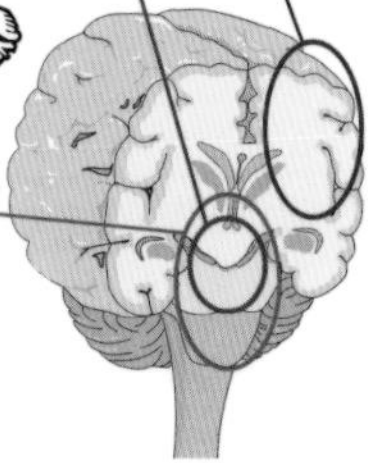

Decerebrate:
(abnormal extension)
Lesion midbrian, brain stem
or pons

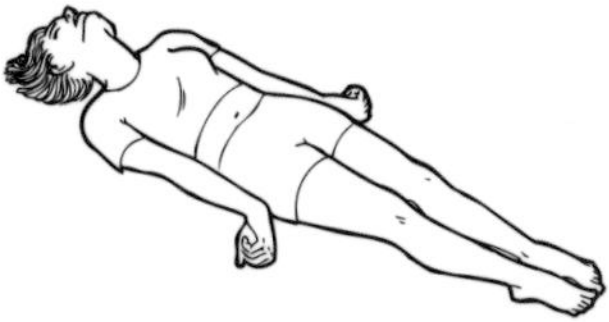

Pupil Gauge (in mm)

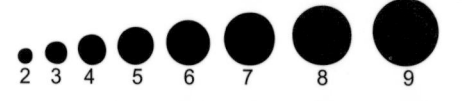

2 3 4 5 6 7 8 9

Fibrinolytic Checklist for Ischemic Stroke

All the "YES" boxes and all the "NO" boxes must be checked before fibrinolytic therapy can be given.

INCLUSION CRITERIA (all must be YES)
☐ Age 18 years or older
☐ Clinical Dx: ischemic stroke causing measurable neuro deficit
☐ Time of symptom onset will be <4.5* hours before fibrinolytic treatment begins (*<3 hours if any: >80 years old, severe stroke [NIHSS >25], on oral anticoagulant, Hx diabetes + prior ischemic stroke)

EXCLUSION CRITERIA (all must be NO)
☐ Prior stroke or head injury within the past 3 months
☐ Intracranial hemorrhage on noncontrast CT
☐ Clinical suspicion subarachnoid bleed, even with normal CT
☐ Arterial puncture within 7 days at a noncompressible site
☐ Multilobar infarction on CT >1/3 cerebral hemisphere
☐ Uncontrolled HTN: systolic BP >185 mm Hg or diastolic BP >110 mm Hg
☐ Evidence of active hemorrhage on exam
☐ Blood glucose <50 mg/dL (2.7 mmol/L)
☐ Hx: previous intracranial bleed, AV malformation, aneurysm, or neoplasm
☐ Active internal bleeding or acute trauma (fracture)
☐ Acute bleeding diathesis, including but not limited to:
   ☐ Platelet count <100,000/mm^3
   ☐ Patient has received heparin within 48 hours and had an elevated aPTT (greater than upper limit of normal for lab)
   ☐ Current use of anticoagulant (e.g., warfarin sodium) with elevated prothrombin time >15 seconds, or INR >1.7

RELATIVE CONTRAINDICATIONS (weigh risks vs. benefits)
☐ Only minor or rapidly improving stroke symptoms
☐ Within 14 days of major surgery or serious trauma
☐ Within 21 days of GI or urinary tract hemorrhage
☐ Recent acute MI within 3 months
☐ Witnessed seizure at stroke onset, with postictal impairments

Los Angeles Prehospital Stroke Screen (LAPSS)

Screening Criteria:

1. Age over 45 years   ❑ Yes ❑ No
2. No prior history of seizure disorder   ❑ Yes ❑ No
3. New neurologic symptoms in last 24 hours   ❑ Yes ❑ No
4. Patient was ambulatory prior to event   ❑ Yes ❑ No
5. Blood glucose between 60–400   ❑ Yes ❑ No
6. Exam (below) reveals only unilateral weakness ❑ Yes ❑ No

Exam: look for obvious asymmetry

	Normal	Right	Left
Facial smile/grimace		Droop	Droop
Grip		Weak grip	Weak grip
		No grip	No grip
Arm weakness		Drifts down	Drifts down
		Falls rapidly	Falls rapidly

7. If "Yes" to all items above, the LAPSS screening criteria are met: **Notify receiving hospital with "code stroke."**

NOTE: The patient may still be experiencing a stroke even if LAPSS criteria are not met.

Cincinnati Prehospital Stroke Scale

Symptoms	Normal	Abnormal
Facial droop	Both sides of face move equally	One side of face does not move as well as other side
Arm drift	Both arms move equally or not at all	One arm drifts compared to the other
Speech	Patient uses correct words with no slurring	Slurred or inappropriate words or mute

NOTE: Any abnormal finding suggests potential stroke.

Poisons and Overdoses

NOTE: This section is not a comprehensive list of of all drugs, poisons, side effects, cautions, or treatments. Before administering any treatments, consult your Poison Center, the product label or insert, your protocols, and/or your On-Line Medical Resource.

Abbreviations Used In This Section

AKA—Common brand®, ™, and "street names"
SE—Common toxic side effects (green text)
Cautions—Primary cautions (red text)
RX—Prehospital care (blue text)

Acids
• *Caustics*

AKA—Rust remover, metal polish.
SE—Pain, GI tract chemical burns, lip burns, vomiting.
RX—Give milk or water, milk of magnesia, egg white, prevent aspiration. Transport patient in sitting position, if possible.
Cautions—Do not induce vomiting.

Acetaminophen
• *Analgesic*

AKA—Tylenol®, APAP.
SE—There may be no symptoms, but acetaminophen is toxic to the liver. N/V, anorexia, RUQ pain, pallor, diaphoresis.
RX—ABCs, IV, ECG, fluids for hypotension. Activated charcoal 1 gm/kg PO or by NG tube, if given within 4 hours of ingestion. Acetylcysteine may be given in ED.

Alkalis • *Caustics*

AKA—Drano®, drain and oven cleaners, bleach.
SE—Pain, GI tract chemical burns, lip burns, vomiting.
RX—Give milk or water, prevent aspiration. Transport patient in sitting position, if possible.
Cautions—Do not induce vomiting.

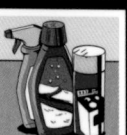

Amphetamines/Stimulants • *Stimulant*

AKA—Methamphetamine, "speed," "crank."
SE—Anxiety, ↑HR, arrhythmias, diaphoresis, seizure, N/V, H/A, CVA, HTN, hyperthermia, dilated pupils, psychosis, suicidal.
RX—ABCs, ECG, IV fluids for hypotension. Activated charcoal 50–100 gm orally. Maintain normal body temp. Benzodiazepine as adjunct.
Cautions—Protect yourself against the violent patient.

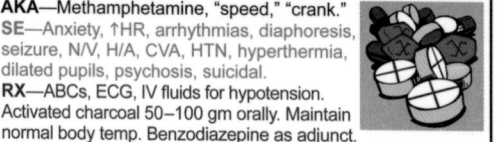

Antidepressants (TCA) • *Mood Elevators*

AKA—Norpramin®, Sinequan®, amitriptyline.
SE—Hypotension, PVCs, cardiac arrhythmias, QRS complex widening, seizures, coma, death.
RX—ABCs, IV, ECG, IV fluids, 1 mEq/kg NaHCO$_3$ IV, intubate and ventilate.
Cautions—Onset of coma and seizures can be sudden. Do not induce vomiting.

Aspirin • *Analgesic*

AKA—Bayer®, ASA, salicylates.
SE—GI bleeding, N/V, LUQ pain, pallor, diaphoresis, shock, tinnitus, ↑RR.
RX—ABCs, IV, ECG, fluids for hypotension. Activated charcoal 1 gm/kg PO.

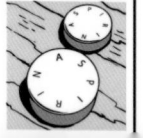

AKA—Phenobarbital, "barbs," "downers."
SE—Weakness, drowsiness, respiratory depression, apnea, hypotension, bradycardia, hypothermia, APE, death.
RX—ABCs, ventilate, IV fluids for hypotension.
Cautions—Protect the patient's airway.

Cannabinoids • *Stimulant/Hallucinogen*

AKA—Marijuana, THC, CBD, "K2", "K3", "Spice"
SE—Euphoria, lethargy, altered perception, confusion, somnolence, difficulty with memory and learning, hallucinations, paranoia, aggressiveness, psychosis, depression, anxiety, nausea, kidney damage, dry mouth, dry or red eyes, hypokalemia, hyperthermia, rhabdomyolsis, cerebral ischemia, seizures, tachycardia, HTN, MI, death.
RX—ABCs, vitals, IV, O_2 prn, EKG. Consider benzodiazepine for agitation, psychosis, seizures. Cool the hyperthermic patient.
Cautions—Protect yourself against the violent patient.

Carbon Monoxide • *Odorless Toxic Gas*

Causes—Any source of incomplete combustion, such as: car exhaust, fire suppression, and stoves.
SE—H/A, dizziness, DOE, fatigue, tachycardia, visual disturbances, hallucinations, cherry red skin color, ↓respirations, N/V, cyanosis, altered mental status, coma, blindness, hearing loss, convulsions.
RX—Remove patient from toxic environment, ABCs, 100% O_2 (check blood glucose), transport. Hyperbaric treatment in severe cases.
Cautions—O_2 sat monitor can give false high reading with CO exposure.

WARNING: Protect yourself from exposure!

Cocaine • *Stimulant/Anesthetic*

AKA—"Coke," "snow," "flake," "crack."
SE—H/A, N/V, ↓RR, agitation, ↑HR, arrhythmias, chest pain, vasoconstriction, AMI, HTN, seizure, vertigo, euphoria, paranoia, vomiting, hyperthermia, tremors, paralysis, coma, dilated pupils, bradycardia, death, APE with IV use.

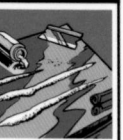

RX—ABCs, IV, ET intubation. Consider: benzodiazepine for seizures, lidocaine for PVCs, nitrates and phentolamine for AMI. Control HTN. Monitor VS and core temp: cool patient if hyperthermic. Minimize sensory stimulation. Consider activated charcoal for oral cocaine ingestion.
Cautions—Protect yourself from the violent patient. A "speedball" is cocaine + heroin. Do not give beta blockers.

Ecstasy/MDMA • *Stimulant/Hallucinogen*

AKA—"XTC," "X," "love drug," "MDMA," "Empathy."
SE—Euphoria, hallucinations, agitation, teeth grinding (use of pacifiers), nausea, hyperthermia, sweating, HTN, tachycardia, renal and heart failure, dilated pupils, seizures, rhabdomyolysis, DIC, APE, CVA, coma, electrolyte imbalance.
RX—ABCs, vitals, ECG, IV, cool patient if hyperthermic, intubate if unconscious, benzodiazepine for seizure and bicarb for myoglobinurea.
Cautions—Do not give beta blockers.

GHB (Gamma-Hydroxybutyrate) • *Depressant*

AKA—"G," "easy lay," "liquid X," "Blue Nitro."
SE—Euphoria, sedation, dizziness, myoclonic jerking, N/V, H/A, coma, bradycardia, apnea.
RX—ABCs, manage airway, ventilate.
Cautions—A common "date rape" drug.

Hallucinogens • Alter Perception

AKA—LSD, psilocybin mushrooms.
SE—Anxiety, hallucinations, panic, disorientation, N/V.
RX—Calm and reassure the patient. Be supportive.
Cautions—Watch for violent and unexpected behavior.

Hydrocarbons • Fuels, Oils

AKA—Gasoline, oil, petroleum products.
SE—Breath odor, SOB, seizures, APE,
coma, bronchospasm.
RX—ABCs, gastric lavage.
Cautions—Do not induce vomiting.

Hydroxocobalamin (Cyanokit®) • Cyanide antidote

RX—Cyanide poisoning: 5 gm diluted in 200 mL NS, LR, D5W,
IV over 15 minutes. May repeat 5 gm IV up to total 10 gm.
Contra—Incompatible with many medications, administer in
separate IV line.
SE— HTN, red skin and body fluid discoloration (urine, tears,
etc), erythema, nausea, headache, reduced lymphocytes,
chromaturia.

Opiates • Narcotic Analgesic

AKA—Dilaudid®, heroin, morphine, codeine, fentanyl.
SE—↓Respirations, apnea, ↓BP, coma, bradycardia, pinpoint
pupils, vomiting, diaphoresis.
RX—ABCs, ventilate, intubate, IV fluids for hypotension,
naloxone 2 mg IV/IO, IM, SQ, ET, IL.
Cautions—Consider other concurrent overdoses.

Poisons

Organophosphates • *Insecticides*

AKA—Malathion®, Diazinon®.
SE—SLUDGE (Salivation, Lacrimation, Urination, Defecation, G-I, Emesis), pinpoint pupils, weakness, bradycardia, sweating, N/V, diarrhea, dyspnea.

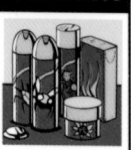

RX—Extricate patient, ABCs. Atropine 1–5 mg IV/IO, IM double doses every 5 minutes until sludge goes away. Start at 2 mg IV/IO, IM for moderate signs and symptoms.
Peds—0.05 mg/kg, every five minutes, until vital signs improve.
Cautions—Protect yourself first! Do not become contaminated.

PCP—Phencyclidine • *Tranquilizer*

AKA—"Peace Pill," "angel dust," "horse tranquilizer."
SE—Nystagmus, disorientation, HTN, hallucinations, catatonia, sedation, paralysis, stupor, mania, tachycardia, dilated pupils, status epilepticus.

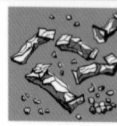

RX—ABCs, vitals, IV, ECG. Consider benzodiazepines.
Cautions—Protect yourself against violent patient. Examine patient for trauma which may have occurred due to anesthetic effect of PCP.

Psychoactive "Bath Salts" • *Stimulant*
(Cathinones, Mephedrone, MDPV, Methylone)

AKA—"Legal high", "Plant food", "Jewelry cleaner", "Flakka"
SE—Agitation, tachycardia, HTN, HA, hyperthermia, euphoria, anxiety, panic attack, psychosis, blurry vision, insomnia, ringing or buzzing in ears, nightmares, depression, self harm, N&V, hyponatremia, acidosis, MI, rhabdomyolysis, seizures, death.
RX—ABCs, vitals, IV, EKG. Consider benzodiazepine for agitation, panic attack, seizures. Cool the hyperthermic patient.
Cautions—Protect yourself against the violent patient

Tranquilizers (major) • *Antipsychotic*

AKA—Haldol®, Navane®, Thorazine®, Compazine®.

SE—EPS, dystonias, painful muscle spasms, respiratory depression, hypotension, torsades de pointes.

RX—Diphenhydramine 25–50 mg IV or deep IM for EPS. ABCs, vitals, ECG. Consider activated charcoal 50–100 gm orally. IV fluids for hypotension. Consider intubation for the unconscious patient.

Cautions—Protect the patient's airway.

Tranquilizers (minor) • *Anxiolytics*

AKA—Valium®, Xanax®, diazepam, midazolam.

SE—Sedation, weakness, dizziness, tachycardia, hypotension, hypothermia, (↓respirations with IV use).

RX—ABCs, monitor vitals; support respirations.

Cautions—Coma usually means some other substance or cause is also involved. OD is almost always in combination with other drugs. Protect the patient's airway.

Emergency Medications

NOTE: This section is not a complete or comprehensive list of all medications. For complete information, please consult the drug product insert, or an appropriate medical resource.

Abbreviations Used In This Section

RX—Primary indications (black text)
Contra—Primary contraindications (red text)
Dosages—(blue/bold text)
SE—Common side effects (green text)
• *Drug Type*—for medications (italic text)
Peds—*Pediatric doses (black italic text)*

Activated Charcoal · *Adsorbent*

RX—**Poisoning/Overdose: 1 gm/kg PO or by NG tube.**
(Mix with water to make a slurry.)
Contra—Contact Poison Center for more advice.
SE—Constipation, black stools, diarrhea.
Peds—*1 gm/kg.*

Adenosine (Adenocard®) · *Antiarrhythmic*

RX—**PSVT: 6 mg (2 mL) IV rapidly over 1–3 seconds**
(flush with 20 mL NS bolus; elevate IV arm). If no effect in
1–2 minutes, **give 12 mg** over 1–3 seconds. **May repeat
12 mg** bolus one more time.
Contra—Second degree or third degree AV block, VT, sick
sinus syndrome.
SE—Transient dysrhythmias, facial flushing, dyspnea, chest
pressure, ↓HR, ↓BP, H/A, nausea, bronchospasm.

NOTE: Adenosine is blocked by the ophyllines; but potentiated
by dipyridamole, carbamazepine.

Peds—*0.1–0.2 mg/kg IV rapidly, IO up to 6 mg. May double
dose if no effect. Maximum: 12 mg/dose.*

NOTE: All doses of Adenosine should be reduced to one-half (50%) in the following clinical settings:

- Hx of cardiac transplantation
- Patients on carbamazepine (Tegretol) and Dipyridamole (Persantine, Aggrenox)
- Administration through any central line

Adenosine may initiate AF with rapid ventricular response in patients with WPWS (Wolff-Parkinson-White syndrome). Use Adenosine with caution in asthma patients as it may cause a reactive airways response in some cases.

Albuterol 0.5% (Ventolin®)   • *Bronchodilator*

RX—Bronchospasm 2° COPD, Asthma: 2.5 mg mixed in 3 mL saline in nebulizer.
Contra—Tachydysrhythmias, HTN, hypokalemia.
SE—Tachydysrhythmias, anxiety, N/V.
Peds—2.5 mg nebulized in 3 mL saline.

Alteplase (Activase® t-PA)   • *Fibrinolytic*

RX—Acute MI (<12 hours old): 100 mg IV over 3 hours. Mix 100 mg in 100 mL sterile water for 1 mg/mL.
Accelerated 1.5-hour infusion:
- Administer **15 mg IV bolus (15 mL) over 2 minutes**
- Then give **0.75 mg/kg (max: 50 mg)** over next 30 minutes
- Followed by **0.5 mg/kg (max: 35 mg)** over next hour

RX—Acute Ischemic Stroke (<3 hours old): 0.9 mg/kg IV (maximum: 90 mg) over **1 hour**.
- Give 10% of the total dose as an IV bolus over 1 minute
- Then give the remaining 90% over the next hour

RX—Acute Pulmonary Embolism: 100 mg IV over 2 hours.

Contra—Any within 3 months: stroke, AV malformation, neoplasm, recent trauma, aneurysm, recent surgery. Active internal bleeding within 21 days; major surgery or trauma within 14 days, aortic dissection, severe HTN, known bleeding disorders, prolonged CPR with thoracic trauma, LP within 7 days, arterial puncture at a non-compressible site. See *ACLS section, Stemi Fibrinolytic Protocol,* for more contraindications.
SE—Reperfusion dysrhythmias, bleeding, shock.

Amiodarone (Cordarone®) • *Antiarrhythmic*

RX—Cardiac Arrest VF/VT: 300 mg IVP. May repeat 150 mg IVP every 3–5 minutes. Maximum: 2,200 mg/24 hours.

RX—Stable Wide Complex Tachycardia:

Rapid infusion:
150 mg IV over 10 minutes. May repeat 150 mg IVP every 10 minutes (mix 150 mg in 100 mL; run at 10 mL/minute or **600 microdrop/minute**). Maximum 2,200 mg/24 hours.

Slow infusion:
360 mg IV over 6 hours (mix 1,000 mg in 500 mL; run at 30 mL/hour or **30 microdrop/minute**).

Maintenance infusion:
540 mg IV over 18 hours (mix 1,000 mg in 500 mL; run at 15 mL/hour or **15 microdrop/minute**).

Contra—Cardiogenic shock, bradycardia, 2°, 3° block; do not use with drugs that prolong QT interval.
SE—Vasodilation, ↓BP, ↓HR, AV block, hepatotoxicity, ↑QTc, VF, VT, 40 day half-life.
Peds—5 mg/kg IV/IO.

Amyl Nitrite • *Cyanide Antidote*

RX—Cyanide Poisoning: Administer vapors from crushed inhalant for 30 seconds, then administer oxygen for 30 seconds, repeat continuously. Consider following with sodium nitrite and sodium thiosulfate.
SE—Hypotension, H/A, nausea.

Aspirin (ASA) • *Antiplatelet*

RX—Acute Myocardial Infarction: 160–325 mg PO (2–4 chewable children's aspirin tablets).
Contra—Allergy. Use caution with: asthma, ulcers, GI bleeding, other bleeding disorders.
SE—GI bleeding.

Atenolol (Tenormin®) • Beta Blocker

RX—VT, VF, Atrial Fib, Atrial Flutter, PSVT, HTN.

RX—Myocardial Salvage for:
- Acute Anterior MI with HTN and Tachycardia
- Large MI <6 hours old
- Refractory Chest Pain or Tachycardia 2° excess sympathetic tone

5 mg IV slowly over 5 minutes. Wait 10 minutes. Then give another 5 mg IV slowly over 5 minutes. If tolerated well, in 10 minutes, give 50 mg, PO dose, titrate to effect.

Contra—CHF, APE, bronchospasm, Hx asthma, ↓HR, 2° or 3° heart block, cardiogenic shock, ↓BP.
SE—↓BP, CHF, bronchospasm, ↓HR, chest pain, H/A, N/V.

NOTE: Calcium blockers may exacerbate side effects.

Atropine Sulfate • Vagolytic

RX—Symptomatic Bradycardia: 0.5–1 mg IVP every 3–5 minutes; up to 0.04 mg/kg total dose, or 3 mg.

RX—Organophosphate or Carbamate Insecticide Poisoning: 1–5 mg IV/IO, IM double doses every 5 minutes until sludge goes away. Start at 2 mg IV/IO, IM for moderate signs and symptoms.
Peds—0.05 mg/kg, every five minutes, until vital signs improve.

RX—Asthma: 0.4–2 mg nebulized in 3 mL saline.
RX—RSI (pediatric): 0.02 mg/kg. Minimum 0.1 mg

Contra—Tachycardia, glaucoma.
SE—Dilated pupils, ↑HR, VT, VF, H/A, dry mouth.

Calcium Chloride 10% • Electrolyte

RX—Calcium Blocker Toxicity, Hypocalcemia with Tetany, Hyperkalemia, Hypermagnesemia: 500–1,000 mg IV over 5–10 minutes.
Contra—VF, digitalis toxicity, hypercalcemia.
SE—↓HR, ↓BP, VF, coronary and cerebral artery spasm, N/V; extravasation causes necrosis.

NOTE: Precipitates with $NaHCO_3$ in IV bag/tubing.

Peds—10–20 mg/kg (0.1–0.2 mL/kg) IV/IO slowly.

Dexamethasone (Decadron®) • Anti-inflammatory

RX—Cerebral Edema, Anaphylaxis, COPD, Spinal Trauma: 10–100 mg IV.
Contra—Uncontrolled infections, TB, ulcers.
Peds—0.25–1 mg/kg IV/IO, IM.

Dextrose 50% • Nutrient

RX—Coma, Hypoglycemia: 25 gm (50 mL) IV.
SE—Tissue necrosis if extravasation occurs.
Contra—Intracerebral bleeding, hemorrhagic CVA.

Diazepam (Valium®) • Anticonvulsant/Sedative

RX—Status Epilepticus: 5–10 mg IV slowly.

RX—Sedation: 5–15 mg IV slowly. (Rectal diazepam: 0.5 mg/kg via 2" rectal catheter. Flush with 2–3 mL of air after administration.)
Contra—Head injury, ↓BP, acute narrow angle glaucoma.
SE—↓Respirations, ↓BP, drowsiness, venous irritation.

NOTE: Overdose may be reversed with flumazenil.

Diphenhydramine (Benadryl®) • Antihistamine

RX—Allergic Reaction, EPS: 25–50 mg IV, or deep IM.
Contra—Asthma, pregnant or lactating females.
SE—Sedation, blurred vision, anticholinergic effects.
Peds—1–2 mg/kg IV/IO slowly, or IM.

Diltiazem (Cardizem®) • Antiarrhythmic

RX—PSVT, Rapid Atrial Fibrillation, Atrial Flutter: 0.25 mg/kg IV/IO slowly over 2 minutes; if no effect in 15 minutes; **0.35 mg/kg IV/IO slowly over 2 minutes.** Drip: 10–15 mg/hour (5 mg/hour for some patients).

Diltiazem (5mg/mL) Bolus Doses in mL	Patient weight in kg					
	50	60	70	80	90	100
1st dose: 0.25 mg/kg →	2.5 mL	3 mL	3.5 mL	4 mL	4.5 mL	5 mL
2nd dose: 0.35 mg/kg →	3.5 mL	4.2 mL	4.9 mL	5.6 mL	6.3 mL	7 mL

[for drip: mix 125 mg (25 mL) in 100 mL IV solution (1 mg/mL) & run at:]

Diltiazem Drip	mg/hour →	5 mg	10 mg	15 mg
	microdrops/minute →	5 gtt	10 gtt	15 gtt

Contra—Second degree or third degree block, ↓BP, sick sinus syndrome, VT; WPW or short PR syndrome with atrial fib or atrial flutter. Do not give with oral beta blockers. Do not give with furosemide in same IV line (flush line first).
SE—Hypotension, bradycardia, H/A, N/V, CHF, dizziness, weakness. Diltiazem ↑serum digoxin levels.

Dopamine (Intropin®) • *Inotrope*

RX—**Hypotension, Bradycardia**: 2–20 mcg/kg/minute.

Low Dose: 2–5 mcg/kg/minute
Medium Dose: 5–10 mcg/kg/minute
High Dose: >10 mcg/kg/minute

Mix 400 mg in 250 mL D5W (1,600 mcg/mL) and run at:

mcg/kg/ min	Patient weight in kg										
	2.5	5	10	20	30	40	50	60	70	80	90	100
2 mcg	–	–	–	1.5	2	3	4	5	5	6	7	8
5 mcg	–	1	2	4	6	8	9	11	13	15	17	19
10 mcg	1	2	4	8	11	15	19	23	26	30	34	38
15 mcg	1.4	3	6	11	17	23	28	34	39	45	51	56
20 mcg	2	4	8	15	23	30	38	45	53	60	68	75

[Microdrops per minute (or mL/hour)]
Contra—↑HR, HTN. ↓dose to 1/10th for patients on MAOIs.
SE—Tachydysrhythmias, VT, VF, HTN, N/V, H/A, ischemia, AMI.

NOTE: Extravasation causes tissue necrosis.

Enalaprilat (Vasotec®)   • *ACE Inhibitor/Antihypertensive*

RX—HTN, Acute MI, CHF: 0.625–1.25 mg IV slowly, (use lower dose if patient is on diuretics). Repeat in 1 hour if no response, then 1.25 mg IV every 6 hours.
Contra—Renal impairment, pregnancy, lactation.
SE—H/A, dizziness, fatigue, ↓LOC, dyspnea, ↓BP, angina.

Epinephrine (Adrenalin®)   • *Sympathomimetic*

RX—Allergic Reaction: 0.3–0.5 mg (0.3–0.5 mL 1:1,000) **SQ.**
Peds—0.01 mg/kg (0.01 mL/kg) SQ—maximum: 0.5 mg.

RX—Anaphylaxis: 0.3–0.5 mg (3–5 mL 1:10,000) **IV.**

RX—Asthma: 0.3–0.5 mg (0.3–0.5 mL 1:1,000) **SQ.**

RX—Bradycardia/Hypotension: 2–10 mcg/minute IV.
(mix 1 mg in 250 mL D5W):

Epinephrine Drip

mcg/minute →	2	3	4	5	6	7	8	9	10
microdrops →	30	45	60	75	90	105	120	135	150

> **RX—Cardiac Arrest: 1 mg IV/IO every 3–5 minutes.**
> **Alternative doses for cardiac arrest:**
>   **High Dose: 0.2 mg/kg IVP every 3–5 minutes.**
>   **Endotracheal Dose: 2–2.5 mg every 3–5 minutes.**

Contra—Tachydysrhythmias, severe coronary artery disease.
SE—Tachydysrhythmias, VT, VF angina, HTN, N/V, anxiety.

Etomidate (Amidate®)   • *Sedative/Hypnotic*

RX—Sedation for RSI: 0.3 mg/kg IV slowly.
Contra—Patient <10 years old, pregnancy, do not use with ketamine, immunosuppression, sepsis, transplant patient.
SE—Apnea, bradycardia, ↓BP, arrhythmias, N/V.

Fentanyl (Sublimaze®) • *Narcotic Analgesic*

RX—Analgesia: 50-100 mcg IV/IM/IO/IN titrated to patient condition and response. Push slow IV over 1-2 minutes, consider dilution for low volumn.
Contra—MAOI use, asthma, myasthenia gravis.
SE—↓LOC,↓BP, N/V, bradycardia, apnea.
Peds—0.5 mcg/kg IV/IO/IM May repeat with 0.5 mcg/kg every 3-5 minutes as needed to a maximum of 4 mcg/kg. Do NOT exceed adult dose. IN 1 mcg/kg.

Flumazenil (Romazicon®) • *Antidote*

RX—Benzodiazepine: 0.2 mg IV/IO; repeat 0.3 mg IV/IO, 0.5 mg IV/IO. If patient not responding after total dose of 5 mg, it is not likely a benzodiazepine overdose.

WARNING: Seizure Risk: Benzodiazepine reversal may result in seizures in some patients. Cyclic antidepressant overdose, status epilepticus, ↑ICP, allergy to benzodiazepines.

SE—Seizure, N/V, agitation, withdrawal. Watch for resedation.
Peds—0.01 mg/kg IV/IO, up to 0.2 mg single dose, repeat every minute, as needed. Maximum total dose: 1 mg.

Furosemide (Lasix®) • *Diuretic*

RX—CHF with Pulmonary Edema, Hypertensive Crisis: 0.5–1 mg/kg IV/IO slowly. Maximum: 2 mg/kg.
Contra—Dehydration, hypokalemia, hepatic coma, anuria.
SE—Hypokalemia, hypotension, dehydration.
Peds—1 mg/kg IV/IO slowly.

Glucagon • ↑*Blood Glucose*

RX—Hypoglycemia: 0.5–1 mg (or Unit) IM, SQ, IV.
Give carbohydrate such as prompt meal, orange juice,
D50%, etc., as soon as the patient is alert and can eat.

**RX—Beta blocker Calcium-Channel OD: 5–10 mg IV over
1 minute**, followed by drip: 1–10 mg/hour.
Peds—0.5–1 mg IV/IO, IM, SQ.

Haloperidol (Haldol®) • *Antipsychotic/Neuroleptic*

**RX—Schizophrenia, mania, psychosis: 2.5-5 mg IV or IM.
May repeat up to 10 mg maximum.**
Contra—Parkinson disease.
SE—Tardive dyskinesia, muscle contractions/tremors,
neuroleptic malignant syndrome, depression, insomnia.
Peds—Ages 3- 7 2 yo: 0.05 IV mg/kg (maximum, 2.5 mg).

Ibutilide (Corvert®) • *Antiarrhythmic*

**RX—Atrial Fibrillation, Atrial Flutter: 1 mg IV slowly over
10 minutes**. For patients <60 kg, give 0.01 mg/kg IV slowly
over 10 minutes. May repeat in 10 minutes.
Contra—Do not give with class 1a antiarrhythmics such as
disopyramide, quinidine, procainamide, or class III drugs such
as amiodarone, sotalol. Use caution with drugs that prolong
the QT interval: phenothiazines, TCAs, and H_1 receptor
antagonists.
SE—PVCs, VT, hypotension, heart block, nausea, H/A,
tachycardia, QT prolongation, torsades, HTN.

Ipratropium .02% (Atrovent®) • *Bronchodilator*

**RX—Bronchospasm, COPD, Asthma: 0.5 mg (2.5 mL "fish")
nebulized (with albuterol), repeat x1.**
Contra—Glaucoma, allergy to soy products or peanuts.
SE—Dry mouth, H/A, cough.
Peds—0.25–0.5 mg.

Ketamine (Ketalar®) • *Anesthetic/Analgesic*

RX—Anesthesia: 2 mg/kg IV every 10–20 minutes (or 10 mg/kg IM every 12–25 minutes).
Contra—Hypertensive crisis, allergy.
SE—HTN, respiratory depression, ↑HR, hallucinations, delirium, confusion.

Ketorolac (Toradol®) • *NSAID Analgesic*

RX—Analgesia: 15–30 mg IV or 30–60 mg IM.
Contra—Kidney disease, labor, allergy to ASA or other NSAIDs.
Use caution in kidney or liver disease, COPD, asthma, ulcers, bleeding disorders, coumadin use, elderly, diabetes.
SE—Nausea, GI bleeding, edema, HTN.

Labetalol (Normodyne®) • *Antihypertensive*

RX—Severe HTN: (choose either bolus loading dose or infusion loading dose):
Bolus Loading: **20 mg IV over 2 minutes.** May double dose every 10 minutes—40 mg, 80 mg, 160 mg, up to 300 mg total dose given.
Infusion Loading Dose: Mix 200 mg (40 mL) in 160 mL of D5W for a concentration of 1 mg/mL. **Start initial infusion at 2 mg/minute and titrate to BP.** May increase up to 6 mg/minute, up to 300 mg total dose infused.

WARNING: Check BP every 5 minutes between doses.

Labetalol Drip (1 mg/mL)			
mg/minute →	2 mg	4 mg	6 mg
microdrops/minute (mL/hour) →	120 gtt	240 gtt	360 gtt

Contra—Asthma, cardiac failure, 2°, 3° block, severe bradycardia, cardiogenic shock, hypotension.
SE—Hypotension, nausea, dizziness, dyspnea.

Lidocaine 2% (Xylocaine®) • *Antiarrhythmic*

RX—Cardiac Arrest VT/VF: 1–1.5 mg/kg IVP; may repeat with 0.5–0.75 mg/kg IVP every 5–10 minutes. Maximum: 3 mg/kg. **ET dose: 2–4 mg/kg.**

RX—VT with Pulse: 1–1.5 mg/kg IVP; then 0.5–0.75 mg/kg every 5–10 minutes up to 3 mg/kg. Start drip ASAP.

RX—PVCs: 0.5–1.5 mg/kg IV; then 0.5–1.5 mg/kg every 5–10 minutes up to 3 mg/kg. Start drip ASAP.

Drip: 1–4 mg/minute. Mix 1 gm in 250 mL D5W and run at:

Lidocaine Drip (4 mg/mL) →	1 mg	2 mg	3 mg	4 mg
microdrops/minute (mL/hr) →	15 gtt	30 gtt	45 gtt	60 gtt

IM Dose: 300 mg IM (4 mg/kg) of 10% solution.
Contra—2°, 3° block, hypotension, Stokes-Adams Syndrome. Reduce maintenance infusion by 50% if patient. is >70 years old, has liver disease, or is in CHF or shock.
SE—Seizure, slurred speech, altered mental status, ↓HR, N/V, tinnitus.

Lisinopril (Prinivil®) • *ACE Inhibitor/Antihypertensive*

RX—Hypertension, AMI: 5–10 mg PO.
Contra—Renal impairment, angioedema, pregnancy, hypovolemia.
SE—H/A, dizziness, fatigue, nausea, ↓BP.

Lorazepam (Ativan®) • *Anticonvulsant/Sedative*

RX—Status Epilepticus: 2–4 mg slowly IV*, or IM.

RX—Anxiety, Sedation: 0.05 mg/kg up to 4 mg IM.
Contra—Acute narrow-angle glaucoma, pregnancy.
SE—Apnea, N/V, drowsiness, restlessness, delirium, ↓BP.

IMPORTANT: Be prepared to ventilate patient.

NOTE: Overdose may be reversed with flumazenil.

***Peds**—0.05–0.1 mg/kg IV/IO* slowly, or IM. Max: 2 mg/dose.*

*For IV/IO use, dilute 1:1 in NS, D5%W, or SW.

Magnesium Sulfate 10% • *Electrolyte*

RX—Cardiac Arrest (Torsades, Hypomagnesemia): 1–2 gm IVP (5–10 gm may be required).

RX—Torsades with a Pulse: 1–2 gm IV over 5–60 minutes (mix in 50 mL D5W). Start drip of 0.5–1 gm/hour and titrate.

RX—Acute MI: 1–2 gm IV over 5–60 minutes (mix in 50 mL D5W). Start drip: 0.5–1 gm/hour; run for up to 24 hours.

RX—Seizures 2° Eclampsia: 1–4 gm IV slowly.

Contra—Renal disease, heart block, hypermagnesemia.
SE—Hypotension, asystole, cardiac arrest, respiratory and CNS depression, flushing, sweating.
Peds—25–50 mg/kg IV/IO over 10–20 minutes. Max: 2 gm.

Meperidine (Demerol®) • *Analgesic*

RX—Analgesia: 50–100 mg IM, SQ or slowly IV.
Contra—Patients receiving MAO inhibitors.
SE—Sedation, apnea, hypotension, ↑ICP, N/V, ↑HR.
Peds—1 mg/kg IV/IO, IM, SQ.

IMPORTANT: Dilute prior to giving IV.

Methylprednisolone (Solu-Medrol®) • *Steroid*

RX—Asthma: 2 mg/kg IV.

RX—Spinal Cord Trauma: 30 mg/kg IV.

Contra—GI Bleed, diabetes, systemic fungal infection.
SE—Euphoria, peptic ulcer, hyperglycemia, hypokalemia.
Peds—Asthma: 2 mg/kg IV/IO, IM.
Peds—Spinal cord injury: 30 mg/kg IV/IO, IM.

Metoprolol (Lopressor®) • Beta Blocker

RX—Atrial Fib, Atrial Flutter, PSVT:
2.5–5 mg every 2–5 minutes. Maximum: 15 mg.

RX—Myocardial Infarction:
5 mg IV slowly over 2–5 minutes, repeated every
5 minutes to a total of 15 mg. Then 50 mg orally, every 6
hours x48 hours, thereafter increased to 100 mg twice a day.
Contra—CHF, APE, bronchospasm, bradycardia,
hypotension, cardiomegaly, thyrotoxicosis, Hx asthma.
SE—↓BP, CHF, bronchospasm, ↓HR, chest pain, H/A, N/V.

NOTE: Calcium blockers may potentiate side effects.

Midazolam (Versed®) • Sedative

RX—Seizures: 2.5 – 5 mg IV/IO, 5 mg IM/intranasal,
repeat every 5 min until seizure stops.

RX—Sedation: combative patient: 5–10 mg IM/intranasal,
repeat every 5 min until not combative.

RX—Procedure sedation: 2.5–5 mg IV/IO or 5 mg IM/
intranasal. May repeat once.
After RSI may repeat every 15 min as needed to maintain
sedation.
Contra—Acute narrow angle glaucoma, shock.
SE—Respiratory depression, apnea, ↓BP, ↓HR, H/A, N/V.
May reverse with flumazenil IV.
Peds—Seizures: 0.1 mg/kg IV/IO may repeat every 5 min
until seizure stops.
Peds—Sedation: 0.1 mg/kg IV/IO (5 mg MAX)
0.2 mg/kg IM/intranasal. May repeat once after 5 min.
RX—Procedures: *0.1 mg/kg IV/IO*
After RSI, may repeat every 15 min as needed to maintain
sedation.
Other procedures 0.1 mg/kg IV/IO MAX 2.5 mg

Milrinone (Primacor®) • *Inotrope/Vasodilator*

RX—CHF: loading dose: 50 mcg/kg over 10 minutes. Use premixed bag or mix 20 mg (20 mL) in 80 mL of D_5W for 200 mcg/mL:

Milrinone Loading Dose

	Patient Weight (kg)					
	50	60	70	80	90	100
Loading dose: 50 mcg/kg	12.5 mL	15 mL	17.5 mL	20 mL	22.5 mL	25 mL
Microdrops/minute for 10 minutes	75 gtt	90 gtt	105 gtt	120 gtt	135 gtt	150 gtt

Maintenance: 0.375–0.75 mcg/kg/minute. Titrate infusion by 0.125 mcg/kg/minute every 15–30 minutes, as needed (maximum daily dose, 1.13 mg/kg/day).

Milrinone Maintenance Infusion

	Patient Weight (kg)					
	50	60	70	80	90	100
0.375 mcg/kg/minute	5.6	6.8	7.9	9	10.1	11.3
0.5 mcg/kg/minute	7.5	9	10.5	12	13.5	15
0.625 mcg/kg/minute	9.4	11.3	13.1	15	16.9	18.8
0.75 mcg/kg/minute	11.3	13.5	15.8	18	20.3	22.5

Microdrops/minute or mL/hour

Contra—Aortic or pulmonary valve disease, impaired renal/hepatic function, pregnancy, lactation. Reduce maintenance infusion for renal impairment.

SE—Hypotension, H/A, angina, dysrhythmias.

Peds—*50–75 mcg/kg IV, IO slowly. Drip: 0.5–0.75 mcg/kg/min.*

Morphine Sulfate • *Analgesic*

RX—Analgesia, Pulmonary Edema: 2–5 mg IV, IM, SQ.
May repeat every 5 minutes up to 10 mg.
Contra—Head injury, exacerbated COPD, depressed
respiratory drive, hypotension, acute abdomen, ↓LOC, labor.

NOTE: Overdose may be reversed with naloxone.

SE—Respiratory depression, ↓BP, ↓LOC, N/V, ↓HR.
***Peds*—0.1–0.2 mg/kg IV/IO, IM, SQ.**

Naloxone (Narcan®) • *Narcotic Antagonist*

**RX—Opiate Overdose; Coma: 0.4–2 mg IV/IO, IM, SQ,
ET, intranasal.** Repeat every 2–3 minutes, if needed, up to
10 mg total dose.
Contra—Do not use on a newborn if the mother is addicted
to narcotics; may cause withdrawal.
SE—Withdrawal symptoms in the addicted patient, APE,
N/V, ↓BP, HTN, seizure.
***Peds*—Suspected opiate overdose**: 0.1 mg/kg IV/IO, IM,
intranasal to a maximum of 4 mg.

Nicardipine (Cardene®) • *Calcium Blocker*

RX—HTN: 5–20 mg/1 hour. Mix 50 mg in 230 mL D5W for
200 mcg/mL. Run at 25–100 mL/hour.

	Nicardipine Drip (200 mcg/mL)			
mg/hour → °	5 mg	10 mg	15 mg	20 mg
mL/hour (gtt/minute)→	25 mL	50 mL	75 mL	100 mL

Contra—Hypotension, aortic stenosis. Caution with renal
failure and hepatic dysfunction.

WARNING: Do not mix with RL.

SE—Edema, hypotension, dizziness, H/A, tachycardia, N/V,
facial flushing, vein irritation: change IV site every 12 hours.

RX—ACS, Angina, Hypertension, CHF with APE:
Contra—↓BP, hypovolemia, intracranial bleeding, aortic stenosis, right ventricle infarction, severe bradycardia or tachycardia, recent use of Viagra®, Cialis® or Levitra®, ↑ICP, tamponade.
SE—HA, hypotension, syncope, tachycardia, flushing.

Nitroglycerin tablets (NITROSTAT®)

0.3–0.4 mg SL, may repeat in 3–5 minutes (maximum: 3 doses).

Nitroglycerin paste (NITRO-BID®)

1–2 cm of paste (6–12 mg) **topically.**

Nitroglycerin spray (NITROLINGUAL®)

1–2 sprays (0.4–0.8 mg) **under the tongue.**

WARNING: Do not shake container.

Nitroglycerin IV (TRIDIL®)

10–20 mcg/minute. Increase by 5–10 mcg/minute every 5 minutes until desired effect. Mix 25 mg in 250 mL D5W (100 mcg/mL) and run at:

Dose in (mcg/min.)		µgtts/minute (or mL/hour)	Dose in (mcg/min.)		µgtts/minute (or mL/hour)
5 mcg	=	3 µgtts/minute	110 mcg	=	66 µgtts/minute
10 mcg	=	6 µgtts/minute	120 mcg	=	72 µgtts/minute
20 mcg	=	12 µgtts/minute	130 mcg	=	78 µgtts/minute
30 mcg	=	18 µgtts/minute	140 mcg	=	84 µgtts/minute
40 mcg	=	24 µgtts/minute	150 mcg	=	90 µgtts/minute
50 mcg	=	30 µgtts/minute	160 mcg	=	96 µgtts/minute
60 mcg	=	36 µgtts/ minute	170 mcg	=	102 µgtts/minute
70 mcg	=	42 µgtts/minute	180 mcg	=	108 µgtts/minute
80 mcg	=	48 µgtts/minute	190 mcg	=	114 µgtts/minute
90 mcg	=	54 µgtts/minute	200 mcg	=	120 µgtts/minute
100 mcg	=	60 µgtts/minute			

NOTE: Use glass IV bottle and non-PVC IV tubing.

Nitroprusside (Nipride®) • *Vasodilator*

RX—Hypertensive crisis, CHF: 0.1–10 mcg/kg/minute.
Start at 0.1 mcg/kg/minute and titrate every 3–5 minutes until desired effect.

Mix 50 mg in 250 mL of D_5W (200 mcg/mL) and run at:

mcg/ kg/ min	Patient Weight (kg)											
	2.5	5	10	20	30	40	50	60	70	80	90	100
0.1 mcg	*	*	0.3	0.6	0.9	1.2	1.5	1.8	2	2.4	2.8	3
0.5 mcg	*	*	1.5	3	4.5	6	7.5	9	10	12	14	15
1 mcg	*	1.5	3	6	9	12	15	18	21	24	27	30
2 mcg	1.5	3	6	12	18	24	30	36	42	48	54	60
4 mcg	3	6	12	24	36	48	60	72	84	96	108	120
8 mcg	6	12	24	48	72	96	120	144	168	192	216	240
10 mcg	7.5	15	30	60	90	120	150	180	210	240	270	300

Microdrops/minute or mL/hour

Contra—Compensatory HTN, hypotension, aortic stenosis, recent use (within 24 hours) of Viagra, Cialis, Levitra.

SE—Hypotension, tachycardia, thiocyanate toxicity, hypoxemia, CO_2 retention, H/A, N/V.

NOTE: Wrap IV bag in foil or other opaque cover.

****Peds*—**For pediatric infusions, see Pediatrics section, Pediatric Medication Infusions chart.

Nitrous Oxide (Nitronox®) • *Analgesic*

RX—Analgesia/Sedation: Give mask to patient and allow to self-administer.

Contra—↓LOC, cyanosis, acute abdomen, shock, ↓BP, pneumothorax, chest trauma, patients who need >50% O_2.

SE—Drowsiness, euphoria, apnea, N/V.

NOTE: Ventilate patient area during use.

Norepinephrine (Levophed®) • *Vasopressor*

RX—Cardiogenic, septic, or neurogenic shock:
0.5–30 mcg/minute. Mix 4 mg in 250 mL of D_5W (16 mcg/mL):

Dose (mcg/minute)	µgtt/minute (or mL/hour)	Dose (mcg/minute)	µgtt/minute (or mL/hour)
0.5 mcg =	2 µgtts/min.	12 mcg =	45 µgtts/min.
1 mcg =	4 µgtts/min.	13 mcg =	49 µgtts/min.
2 mcg =	8 µgtts/min.	14 mcg =	53 µgtts/min.
3 mcg =	11 µgtts/min.	15 mcg =	56 µgtts/min.
4 mcg =	15 µgtts/min.	16 mcg =	60 µgtts/min.
5 mcg =	19 µgtts/min.	17 mcg =	64 µgtts/min.
6 mcg =	23 µgtts/min.	18 mcg =	68 µgtts/min.
7 mcg =	26 µgtts/min.	19 mcg =	71 µgtts/min.
8 mcg =	30 µgtts/min.	20 mcg =	75 µgtts/min.
9 mcg =	34 µgtts/min.	25 mcg =	94 µgtts/min.
10 mcg =	38 µgtts/min.	30 mcg =	113 µgtts/min.
11 mcg =	41 µgtts/min.		

Contra—Hypovolemia (unless as a temporary measure until volume can be replaced); mesenteric or peripheral vascular thrombosis; ischemic heart disease.

SE—Tachydysrhythmias, VT, VF, HTN, N/V, AMI, ischemia; decreased renal perfusion; Ø urine output.

NOTE: Extravasation causes tissue necrosis—give phentolamine (Regitine®) in the area of the infiltrate: 5–10 mg diluted in 10–15 mL of saline.

Peds—0.1–2 mcg/kg/minute and titrate to effect.

Ondansetron (Zofran®) • *Antinauseant*

RX—Nausea and Vomiting: 4–8 mg IV slowly, or IM, or 8 mg PO.
Contra—Hypersensitivity to dolasetron, granisetron. May precipitate with bicarb.
SE—H/A, diarrhea, FV, dizziness, pain, seizure, EPS, QT prolongation.
Peds—0.1 mg/kg slow IV/IO or IM. Maximum: 4 mg.

Oxytocin (Pitocin®) • *↑Uterine Contractions*

RX—Postpartum Hemorrhage: 10 units IM after placenta delivers. Or mix 10–40 units in 1,000 mL balanced salt solution and titrate to control uterine bleeding.
Contra—Rule out multiple fetuses before administration.
SE—HTN, dysrhythmias, N/V, anaphylactic reaction.

Pancuronium *(Pavulon®)* • *Paralytic*

RX—Paralysis to Facilitate Tracheal Intubation: 0.04–0.1 mg/kg IVP (onset 3 minutes; recovery: 30–45 minutes). Maintenance: 0.01 mg/kg every 60 minutes.
Contra—1st trimester pregnancy; use reduced dose in newborns, myasthenia gravis.
SE—Apnea, prolonged paralysis, tachycardia, hypotension, hypertension.

Phenobarbital (Luminal®) • *Anticonvulsant*

RX—Status Epilepticus: 10–20 mg/kg IV slowly, or IM.
Contra—Porphyria, pulmonary or hepatic dysfunction.
SE—Respiratory depression, hypotension, coma, N/V.
Peds—10–20 mg/kg IV/IO slowly, or IM. May repeat.

Phenylephrine (Neosynephrine®)   • *Pressor*

RX—PSVT: 0.5 mg IV in 20–30 seconds.

RX—Hypotension: 0.1–0.5 mg slowly every
10–15 minutes, as necessary, to obtain BP.

Maintenance infusion: 40–60 mcg/minute.

Mix 10 mg in 500 mL of D_5W (20 mcg/mL), and run at:

Phenylephrine Drip (20 mcg/mL)

mcg/minute	40 mcg	45 mcg	50 mcg	55 mcg	60 mcg
microdrops/minute (mL/hour)	120 gtt	135 gtt	150 gtt	165 gtt	180 gtt

Contra—Severe HTN, VT, mesenteric or peripheral ischemia.
Use caution in patients with heart block, hyperthyroidism,
bradycardia, severe arteriosclerosis.

SE—H/A, seizure, weakness, CVA, chest pain, bradycardia,
HTN, dysrhythmias, restlessness, respiratory distress.

WARNING: If extravasation occurs: stop infusion; inject 5–10
mg of phentolamine SQ mixed in 10–15 mL of NS.

Potentiated by TCAs, atropine, oxytocics, and MAOIs.
Antagonized by diuretics, α- and β-blockers, phenothiazines.

Phenytoin (Dilantin®)   • *Anticonvulsant*

RX—Seizures: 10–20 mg/kg IV/IO slowly
(maximum: 50 mg/minute).

Contra—Hypoglycemic seizures (give glucose), ↓HR,
second degree or third degree heart block, impaired hepatic
or renal function, ↓BP, hyperglycemia.

SE—Lethargy, H/A, irritability, restlessness, vertigo,
hypotension, bradycardia.

WARNING: Caustic to veins. Use central line if possible.
Flush line after each dose.

Peds—15–20 mg/kg over 30 minutes. Maximum: 1 gm.

Procainamide (Pronestyl®)   • *Antiarrhythmic*

RX—Cardiac arrest VF/VT: 50-mg/minute IV drip (maximum dose, 17 mg/kg).

RX—Atrial fibrillation, VT, PSVT with WPW: 20 mg/minute IV until dysrhythmia is converted, hypotension or QRS/QT widening develops, or 17 mg/kg has been given.

Drip: 1–4 mg/minute. Mix 1 g in 250 mL of D_5W and run at:

Procainamide Drip

mg/minute	1 mg	2 mg	3 mg	4 mg
microdrops/minute (mL/hour)	15 gtt	30 gtt	45 gtt	60 gtt

Contra—2° and 3° AV block, torsades de pointes, lupus, digitalis toxicity, myasthenia gravis.

SE—PR, QRS, and QT widening; AV block; cardiac arrest; hypotension; seizure; N/V.

***Peds**—15 mg/kg IV, IO over 30–60 minutes.*
***Peds Drip**—20–80 mcg/kg/minute.*

Promethazine (Phenergan®)   • *Antiemetic/Sedative*

RX—Nausea and Vomiting: 12.5 –25 mg IV, IM, or 25 mg PO.

RX—Sedation: 25 – 50 mg IV, IM, PO.

Contra—<2 years old, allergy to antihistamines and phenothiazines, lactating females, MAOI use, COPD, HTN, pregnancy.

WARNING: May cause respiratory depression, severe tissue injury, gangrene.

SE—Drowsiness, viscous bronchial secretions, urinary urgency, EPS, confusion, ↑HR, ↓HR.

***Peds—Nausea and Vomiting**: 0.25 –1 mg/kg IV/IO, PO.*
***Peds—Sedation**: 0.5 –1 mg/kg IV/IO.*

Propofol (Diprivan®)   • *Anesthetic*

RX—Anesthesia: 2–2.5 mg/kg IV over 1 minute until onset of anesthesia.

Maintenance: 100–200 mcg/kg/minute.
Reduce dose for elderly, debilitated, or neurosurgical patient.

RX—Sedation: 100–150 mcg/kg/minute over 3–5 minutes, followed by maintenance infusion of 25–75 mcg/kg/minute.

RX—ICU sedation in the intubated patient: 5 mcg/kg/minute over at least 5 minutes. May increase by 5–10 mcg/kg/minute, every 5–10 minutes until desired level of sedation. Maintenance infusion: 5–50 mcg/kg/minute may be required. Maximum dose: 150 mcg/kg/minute (some may require higher dose).

Contra—↑ ICP, impaired cerebral circulation, lipid metabolism disorders, respiratory, renal, circulatory, or hepatic disease.

SE—Apnea, hypotension, N/V, pain at IV site, jerking, H/A, bradycardia, HTN, fever. Reduce dose if patient has received large doses of narcotics.

Use 100-mL vial (10 mg/mL) and run at:

mcg/kg/min	35	40	45	50	55	60	65	70	75	80	90	100
5 mcg	1.05	1.2	1.35	1.5	1.65	1.8	1.95	2.1	2.25	2.4	2.7	3
10 mcg	2.1	2.4	2.7	3	3.3	3.6	3.9	4.2	4.5	4.8	5.4	6
20 mcg	4.2	4.8	5.4	6	6.6	7.2	7.8	8.4	9	9.6	10.8	12
30 mcg	6.3	7.2	8.1	9	9.9	10.8	11.7	12.6	13.5	14.4	16.2	18
40 mcg	8.4	9.6	10.8	12	13.2	14.4	15.6	16.8	18	19.2	21.6	24
50 mcg	10.5	12	13.5	15	16.5	18	19.5	21	22.5	24	27	30
60 mcg	12.6	14.4	16.2	18	19.8	21.6	23.4	25.2	27	28.8	32.4	36
70 mcg	14.7	16.8	18.9	21	23.1	25.2	27.3	29.4	31.5	33.6	37.8	42
80 mcg	16.8	19.2	21.6	24	26.4	28.8	31.2	33.6	36	38.4	43.2	48
90 mcg	18.9	21.6	24.3	27	29.7	32.4	35.1	37.8	40.5	43.2	48.6	54
100 mcg	21	24	27	30	33	36	39	42	45	48	54	60
150 mcg	31.5	36	40.5	45	49.5	54	58.5	63	67.5	72	81	90
200 mcg	42	48	54	60	66	72	78	84	90	96	108	120
250 mcg	52.5	60	67.5	75	82.5	90	97.5	105	113	120	135	150
300 mcg	63	72	81	90	99	108	117	126	135	144	162	180

Microdrops per minute or mL/hour

Peds—1–2.5 mg/kg IV over 1–2 minutes.
Drip: 100–300 mcg/kg/minute.

Reteplase (Retavase®) • *Fibrinolytic*

**RX—Acute MI (<12 hours old): 10 units IV over 2 minutes.
Repeat dose in 30 minutes.** (Flush with NS before and after.)
Contra—Active internal bleeding. Any within 3 months: stroke,
AV malformation, neoplasm, aneurysm, recent trauma, recent
surgery. Bleeding disorders, LP within 7 days. See *ACLS
section, Stemi Fibrinolytic Protocol* for more contraindications.
SE—Dysrhythmias, bleeding, ↓BP, shock, fever, allergy.

Rocuronium (Zemuron®) • *Paralytic*

RX—Paralysis to facilitate tracheal intubation:
- 0.6–1.2 mg/kg IVP (onset: 1–3 minutes; recovery:
  30 minutes). Maintenance: 0.1–0.2 mg/kg every
  12 minutes.

Contra—Caution if impaired hepatic or respiratory function or
if severe obesity.

SE—Bronchospasm, dysrhythmias, hypotension, HTN.

Sodium Bicarbonate 8.4% • *Alkalinizer*

RX—Cardiac Arrest with Good Ventilation: 1 mEq/kg IV,
(1 mL/kg) followed by 0.5 mEq/kg every 10 minutes.

**RX—Hyperkalemia; OD of: Tricyclic, Phenobarbital,
Diphenhydramine, ASA, Cocaine: 1 mEq/kg IV.**
SE—Metabolic alkalosis, ↓K+, fluid overload.

WARNING: Tissue necrosis may occur with extravasation.

Contra—Alkalosis, hypocalcemia, CHF, hypovolemia,
hypernatremia.

Streptokinase (Streptase®)   • *Fibrinolytic*

RX—Acute MI (<12 hours old): 1,500,000 units infused over 60 minutes.

RX—Pulmonary Embolism: 250,000 units over 30 minutes. Follow with infusion of 100,000 units/hour.
Contra—Active internal bleeding within 21 days. Surgery or trauma within 14 days. Aortic dissection, severe HTN, bleeding disorders, prolonged CPR with thoracic trauma, lumbar puncture within 7 days, arterial puncture at a noncompressible site. Any within 3 months: stroke, AV malformation, neoplasm, aneurysm, recent trauma, recent surgery. Streptokinase use within past 2 years.
SE—Reperfusion dysrhythmias, bleeding, shock, H/A, hypotension, allergic reaction, intracranial hemorrhage, N/V, fever.

Succinylcholine (Anectine®)   • *Paralytic*

RX—Paralysis to Facilitate ET Intubation: 1–2 mg/kg IV/IO (onset: 1 minute; recovery: 4–6 minutes). (IM dose: 3–4 mg/kg, maximum: 150 mg [onset: 2–3 minutes].)
Contra—Acute narrow angle glaucoma, penetrating eye injuries, burns >8 hours, massive crush injury.
SE—Apnea, malignant hyperthermia, dysrhythmias, ↓HR, HTN, ↓BP, cardiac arrest, ↑K⁺, ↑intraocular pressure.

Peds—Smaller children: 2 mg/kg; older children and adolescents: 1 mg/kg.

WARNING: Use caution in children and adolescents. May cause hyperkalemia, arrhythmias, cardiac arrest.

Tenecteplase (TNKase) • Fibrinolytic

RX—Acute MI (<12 hours old): 30–50 mg IVP over 5 seconds.
(For bolus: mix 50 mg vial in 10 mL SW [5 mg/mL] and give:)

Patient weight in kg →	50	60	70	80	90	100
Bolus dose in mL →	6 mL	7 mL	8 mL	9 mL	10 mL	10 mL

Contra—Previous hemorrhagic stroke; other CVA within 1 year, intracranial CA, internal bleeding, aortic dissection.

NOTE: See ACLS section, Stemi Fibrinolytic Protocol, for more contraindications.

SE—Intracranial hemorrhage, dysrhythmias, bleeding, ↓BP, shock, CHF.

Thiamine (Vitamin B₁) • Nutrient

RX—Co-administration with D50%W in patients suspected of malnutrition or thiamine deficiency (starvation, severe alcoholism): **100 mg slow IV or IM.**
Contra—Hypersensitivity.
SE—N/V, hypotension, rash, warm sensation, anaphylaxis.

Vecuronium (Norcuron®) • Paralytic

RX—Paralysis/ET Intubation: 0.1 mg/kg IVP
(onset: 2–3 minutes; recovery: 30–45 minutes).
Maintenance: 0.01–0.05 mg/kg.
Contra—Newborns, neuromuscular disease.
SE—Apnea, weakness, bronchospasm.
Peds—0.1 mg/kg IV/IO.

Verapamil (Isoptin®) • Antiarrhythmic

RX—PSVT, Rapid Atrial Fibrillation, Atrial Flutter:
2.5–5 mg IV slowly over 2–3 minutes. May repeat with 5–10 mg every 15–30 minutes. Maximum dose: 20 mg.
Contra—Wide-complex tachycardia, heart failure, impaired ventricular function, hypotension, shock, sick sinus syndrome, second degree or third degree block, AF with WPW or LGL, IV beta blocker use, children <1 year old.

SE—Hypotension, AV block, bradycardia, asystole.
Peds—0.1–0.3 mg/kg IV/IO slowly. Maximum: 5 mg/initial dose.
May give second dose in 30 minutes, up to 10 mg.

Notes

IV fluid rates in drops/minute

Drip Set	10	12	15	20	60*
30 mL/hour	5	6	8	10	30
60 mL/hour	10	12	15	20	60
100 mL/hour	17	20	25	33	100
200 mL/hour	33	40	50	67	200
300 mL/hour	50	60	75	100	300
400 mL/hour	67	80	100	133	400
500 mL/hour	83	100	125	167	500
1,000 mL/hour	167	200	250	333	1,000

**Standard "microdrip" IV tubing has 60 gtt/mL.
A normal "TKO" or "KVO" rate is 8–15 mL/hour.
(Note that with a microdrip IV set, mL/hour = drops/minute).

Notes

Pulse Oximetry

Ranges	Prehospital Care
Normal: 95–99%	
Mild hypoxia: 91–94%	Give oxygen
Moderate hypoxia: 86–90%	Give 100% oxygen
Severe hypoxia: ≤85%	100% oxygen, ventilate

❖ Falsely low SpO_2 readings may be caused by:
  - Cold extremities
  - Hypothermia
  - Hypovolemia
❖ Falsely high SpO_2 readings may be caused by:
  - Anemia
  - Carbon monoxide poisoning
❖ All starting readings must be interpreted in ratio to patient hemoglobin level.

NOTE: If in doubt, give oxygen in spite of a normal SpO_2.

O_2 Tank Capacities

Tank	Capacity	15 Lpm	10 Lpm	6 Lpm	2 Lpm
C	240 L	16 min.	24 min.	40 min.	2 hr.
D	360 L	24 min.	36 min.	1 hr.	3 hr.
E	625 L	41 min.	1:02 hr.	1:44 hr.	5:12 hr.
M	3,000 L	3:20 hr.	5:00 hr.	8:20 hr.	25 hr.
G	5,300 L	5:53 hr.	8:50 hr.	14:43 hr.	44:10 hr.
H	6,900 L	7:40 hr.	11:30 hr.	19:10 hr.	57:30 hr.

Pediatric Cardiac Arrest

Shout for help, activate emergency response, begin CPR, give O_2, attach defibrillator.

VF or Pulseless VT	**Asystole/PEA**

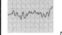 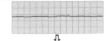

VF or Pulseless VT

⇩

✓ Defibrillate 2 J/kg
Continue CPR immediately
(2 minutes of 15:2*)
Obtain IV or IO access

⇩

Still VF/VT? ✓ Shock 4 J/kg
Continue CPR x2 minutes
Epinephrine IV/IO 0.01 mg/kg
(1:10,000, 0.1 mL/kg)
every 3–5 minutes *OR:*
ET: 0.1 mg/kg (1:1,000, 0.1 mL/kg)
Consider advanced airway
(ET Tube, supraglottic airway)
Ventilate 10 breaths/minute
with continuous compressions
Use waveform capnography:
If PETCO₂ <10, improve CPR.

⇩

Still VF/VT? ✓ Shock ≥4 J/kg
(maximum 10 J/kg or adult dose)
Continue CPR (2 minutes)
Amiodarone 5 mg/kg IV/IO;
may repeat twice.
❖**Identify and Treat Causes**

⇩

Still VF/VT? ✓ Shock ≥4 J/kg
(maximum 10 J/kg or adult dose)
Continue CPR (2 minutes)
Verify paddle position/contact

⇩

If ROSC (pulse, BP, PETCO₂
≥40 mm Hg), provide
post cardiac care.

Asystole/PEA

⇩

Continue CPR immediately
(2 minutes of 15:2*)
Obtain IV or IO access
Epinephrine IV/IO: 0.01 mg/kg
(1:10,000, 0.1 mL/kg)
every 3–5 minutes *OR:*
*ET: 0.1 mg/kg
(1:1,000; 0.1 mL/kg)*
Consider advanced airway
(ET Tube, supraglottic airway)
Ventilate 10 breaths/minute
with continuous compressions
Use waveform capnography:
If PETCO₂ <10, improve CPR.

VF/VT? —Start VF/VT
algorithm on left.
Otherwise: CPR (2 minutes);
repeat **Epinephrine** above.

❖**Identify and Treat Causes**
- Hypoxia
- Acidosis
- Hypovolemia
- Toxins
- Hypoglycemia
- Hyper/Hypokalemia
- Hypothermia
- Pulmonary Thrombosis
- Tension Pneumothorax
- Cardiac Tamponade
- Coronary Thrombosis

*After advanced airway,
10 breaths/minute.

108

Pediatric Bradycardia
(with a pulse, but symptomatic)

Treat Reversible Causes❖
maintain airway, administer O₂, ventilate as needed,
attach ECG, assess BP, SaO₂,
start IV or IO, 12-lead ECG (but do not delay treatment)
⇩
Severe cardiorespiratory compromise?
(altered mental status, hypotension, shock)

YES

Start CPR if HR <60/minute in spite
of good oxygenation and ventilation
Oxygenate, ventilate
**Still Bradycardic after 2 minutes
of CPR?** *(If not)*
⇩
Check airway, O₂ source,
ventilation adequacy.
Epinephrine IV/IO: 0.01 mg/kg
(1:10,000, 0.1 mL/kg)
every 3–5 minutes OR:
ET: 0.1 mg/kg (1:1,000; 0.1 mL/kg)
⇩
Atropine 0.02 mg/kg IV/IO
*(OR: ET: 0.04–0.06 mg/kg) for increased
vagal tone or primary AV block
(minimum dose: 0.1 mg; maximum
single dose: 0.5 mg)
[May repeat x1: maximum
total dose: 1 mg]*
Consider Pacing
Treat Reversible Causes❖
⇩
If arrest develops See *Peds Section,
Pediatric Cardiac Arrest*

NO

Support ABCs,
O₂, **Observe,
Consult with expert**

❖Reversible Causes:
• Hypoxia
• Acidosis
• Hypovolemia
• Toxins
• Hypoglycemia
• Hyper/Hypokalemia
• Hypothermia
• Pulmonary
  Thrombosis
• Tension
  Pneumothorax
• Cardiac Tamponade
• Coronary
  Thrombosis

NOTE: Pediatric
bradycardia is often
the result of hypoxia.

Pediatric Tachycardia
(with poor perfusion)

Treat Reversible Causes❖ (below)
Maintain airway, administer O₂, ventilate as needed,
attach ECG, assess BP, SaO₂, Start IV or IO,
12-lead ECG (but do not delay treatment)

QRS DURATION?

**Narrow QRS
≤0.09 seconds**

**Wide QRS?
>0.09 seconds**

Probably Sinus Tach if:

Compatible history?
Normal P waves?
Variable R-R and normal PR?
Infant HR <220/minutes?
Child HR <180/minutes?
⇩
Treat Reversible Causes❖
(below)

Possibly SVT if:

Hx abrupt rate changes?
Absent/abnormal P waves?
HR not variable?
Infant HR ≥220/minute?
Child HR ≥180/minute?
⇩
Consider vagal maneuvers
(do not delay treatment)
⇩
Adenosine 0.1 mg/kg IVP/IO
(6 mg maximum dose)
May repeat with 0.2 mg/kg
(12 mg maximum dose) **OR:**
⇩
**Synchronized
cardioversion**
(0.5–1.0 J/kg; may increase
to 2 J/kg if initial dose fails;
sedate if possible, but do
not delay cardioversion)
⇩
Consult expert

❖Identify and Treat Causes
• Hypoxia
• Acidosis
• Hypovolemia
• Toxins
• Hypoglycemia
• Hyper/Hypokalemia
• Hypothermia
• Pulmonary Thrombosis
• Tension Pneumothorax
• Cardiac Tamponade
• Coronary Thrombosis

Go to next page

Wide QRS? >0.09 seconds

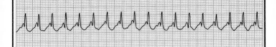

Unstable Patient
(Hypotension, Shock, AMS)

Possible V-Tach
⤳ Synchronized Cardioversion
0.5 J–1.0 J/kg; may increase
to 2 J/kg if initial dose fails
(sedate if possible, but do not
delay cardioversion)
⇩
Consult with expert

Stable Patient

Hemodynamically stable?
Consider Adenosine
0.1 mg/kg IVP/IO
(6 mg maximum dose)
if regular monomorphic QRS
⇩
Consult expert
⇩
Either:
**Amiodarone 5 mg/kg IV over
20–60 minutes**
OR:
**Procainamide 15 mg/kg IV
over 30–60 minutes**

Pediatric Medications

Age	Preterm	Term	6 mos	1 yr	3 yrs.	6 yrs.	8 yrs.	10 yrs.	11 yrs.	12 yrs.	14 yrs.
Weight (pounds)	3	7.5	15	22	33	44	55	66	77	88	99
Weight (kilograms)	1.5	3.5	7	10	15	20	25	30	35	40	45
Length (inches)	16"	21"	26"	31"	39"	46"	50"	54"	57"	60"	64"
Length (cm)	41	53	66	79	99	117	127	137	145	152	163
Heart Rate	140	125	120	120	110	100	90	90	85	85	80
Respirations	40–60	40–60	24–36	22–30	20–26	20–24	18–22	18–22	16–22	16–22	14–20
Systolic BP	50–60	60–70	60–120	65–125	100	100	105	110	110	115	115
ET Tube Size (mm)	2.5, 3.0	3.5	3.5	4.0	4.5	5.5	6.0	6.5	6.5	7.0	7.0
Suction catheter size	5–6 Fr	8 Fr	8 Fr	8 Fr	8 Fr	10 Fr	10 Fr	10 Fr	10 Fr	10 Fr	10 Fr
Defibrillation: 2 J/kg (initial)	3 J	7 J	14 J	20 J	30 J	40 J	50 J	60 J	70 J	80 J	90 J
4 J/kg (repeat)	6 J	14 J	28 J	40 J	60 J	80 J	100 J	120 J	140 J	160 J	180 J
8 J/kg (repeat)	12 J	28 J	56 J	80 J	120 J	160 J	200 J	240 J	280 J	320 J	360 J
10 J/kg (repeat)	15 J	35 J	70 J	100 J	150 J	200 J	250 J	300 J	350 J	360 J	360 J
Cardioversion: 0.5–2 J/kg	1–3 J	2–7 J	4–14 J	5–20 J	8–30 J	10–40 J	13–50 J	15–60 J	18–70 J	20–80 J	23–90 J
Fluid challenge 20 mL/kg IV/IO [Neonates:10 mL/kg]	15 mL [10 mL/kg]	35 mL [10 mL/kg]	140 mL	200 mL	300 mL	400 mL	500 mL	600 mL	700 mL	800 mL	900 mL

Age	Preterm	Term	6 mos	1 yr	3 yrs.	6 yrs.	8 yrs.	10 yrs.	11 yrs.	12 yrs.	14 yrs.
Weight	1.5 kg	3.5 kg	7 Kg	10 kg	15 kg	20 kg	25 kg	30 kg	35 kg	40 kg	45 kg
Amiodarone (50 mg/mL) 5 mg/kg IV/IO	0.15 mL	0.35 mL	0.7 mL	1 mL	1.5 mL	2 mL	2.5 mL	3 mL	3.5 mL	4 mL	4.5 mL
Atropine (0.1 mg/mL) 0.02 mg/kg IV/IO	1 mL	1 mL	1.4 mL	2 mL	3 mL	4 mL	5 mL	6 mL	7 mL	8 mL	9 mL
Dextrose (D50%W) 0.5 gm/kg IV/IO [use D25%W for infant]	3 mL [D25%]	7 mL [D25%]	14 mL [D25%]	20 mL [D25%]	15 mL	20 mL	25 mL	30 mL	35 mL	40 mL	45 mL
Diazepam (5 mg/mL) 0.1–0.3 mg/kg slow IV/IO	0.03–0.09 mL	0.07–0.21 mL	0.14–0.42 mL	0.2–0.6 mL	0.3–0.9 mL	0.4–1.2 mL	0.5–1.5 mL	0.6–1.8 mL	0.7–2.1 mL	0.8–2.4 mL	0.9–2.7 mL
Epi 1:10,000 (0.1 mg/mL) 0.01 mg/kg IV/IO	0.15 mL	0.35 mL	0.7 mL	1 mL	1.5 mL	2 mL	2.5 mL	3 mL	3.5 mL	4 mL	4.5 mL
ET Epinephrine 1:1,000 (1 mg/mL) 0.1 mg/kg ET (& 2nd dose IV/IO)	0.15 mL	0.35 mL	0.7 mL	1 mL	1.5 mL	2 mL	2.5 mL	3 mL	3.5 mL	4 mL	4.5 mL
Etomidate (2 mg/mL) 0.3 mg/kg IV/IO	0.2 mL	0.5 mL	1 mL	1.5 mL	2.3 mL	3 mL	3.8 mL	4.5 mL	5.3 mL	6.8 mL	6.8 mL
Morphine (1 mg/mL) 0.1 mg/kg IV/IO, IM	0.15 mL	0.35 mL	0.7 mL	1 mL	1.5 mL	2 mL	2.5 mL	3 mL	3.5 mL	4 mL	4.5 mL
Naloxone (0.4 mg/mL) 0.1 mg/kg IV/IO, IM, SQ	0.4 mL	0.9 mL	1.8 mL	2.5 mL	3.8 mL	5 mL	5 mL	5 mL	5 mL	5 mL	5 mL
Succinylcholine (20 mg/mL) 1 mg/kg IV/IO [infant: 2 mg/kg]	0.15 mL [2 mg/kg]	0.35 mL [2 mg/kg]	0.7 mL [2 mg/kg]	1 mL [2 mg/kg]	0.75 mL	1 mL	1.25 mL	1.5 mL	1.75 mL	2 mL	2.3 mL

Pediatric Trauma Score

	+2	+1	-1	Score
Patient Size	>20 kg	10–20 kg	<10 kg	
Airway	Normal	Maintainable without invasive procedures	Not maintainable NEEDS invasive procedures	
CNS	Awake	Obtunded	Comatose	
Systolic BP (or pulse)	>90 (radial)	50–90 (femoral)	<50 mm Hg (no pulse)	
Open wounds	None	Minor	Major or Penetrating	
Skeletal	None	Closed fracture	Open/Multiple Fracture	
			Total =	

>12 = <1% mortality, minimal or no injury
≤8 = Critical injury: transport to Pediatric Trauma Center
4 = Predicts 50% mortality
<1 = Predicts >98% mortality

Intraosseous Infusion

NOTE: Most medications, blood products, or solutions that can be given IV, can be given IO.

1. **Locate anterior medial (flat) surface of tibia, 2 cm below tibial tuberosity, below growth plate** (other sites: distal anterior femur, medial malleolus, iliac crest).

2. **Prep area with iodine.**

3. Advance IO needle at 90° angle through skin, fascia, and bone with constant pressure and twisting motion. Direct needle slightly away from epiphyseal plate.

4. **A popping sensation will occur** (and a lack of resistance) **when you have reached the marrow space.**

5. **Attempt to aspirate marrow** (you may or may not get marrow).

6. **Infuse fluids and check for infiltration.** Discontinue if site becomes infiltrated with fluid or medications; apply manual pressure to site followed by a pressure dressing.

7. Secure IO needle, tape in place and attach to IV pump.

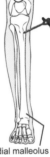

medial malleolus

Pediatric Emergencies—General Assessment

Airway: Look for obstruction, drooling, trauma.
Breathing: Retractions? Respiratory rate? Good air movement?
Circulation: Heart rate? Capillary refill?

WARNING: Bradycardia means hypoxia. Ventilate!

Pediatrics

Pediatric Assessment

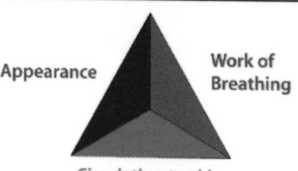

The Pediatric Assessment Triangle

Used with permission of the American Academy of Pediatrics, *Pediatric Education for Prehospital Professionals*, Copyright American Academy of Pediatrics, 2000.

Appearance

Mental status

Muscle tone

Body position

Breathing

Visible movement

Work of breathing (normal/increased)

Circulation

Color

Abbreviations Used on This Page

HX—History, Signs, and Symptoms (black text)
Key Symptoms and Findings (green text)
➕—Prehospital Treatment (blue text with yellow background)
Cautions—Primary Cautions (red text)

Mental Status: Is Child Acting Normally?

HX—Present illness/onset, intake, GI habits. Perform Exam:
Fever? Skin color? Other findings?

➕—**Children in shock need aggressive treatment**.
- Ventilate. Reassess the airway, especially during transport
- Check CBG, consider Naloxone
- IV fluid challenge (20 mL/kg—repeat if necessary)
  Do not wait for BP to drop—hypotension is a late sign
- Rapid transport to a pediatric intensive care facility

Cautions—Not every seizure with fever is a febrile seizure.

- ✔ Consider meningitis, especially in children <2 years old (check for a rash that does not blanch).
- ✔ Early signs of sepsis are subtle: grunting respirations, temperature instability, hypoglycemia, poor feeding, etc.
- ✔ Consider toxins.

Asthma

HX—Difficulty breathing, shortness of breath, coughing, wheezing, decreased or absent lung sounds, tripod positioning, use of accessory muscles, cyanosis, fever/chills, sputum color, urticaria, skin temp, lethargy. Onset, duration and progression, triggers, response to home treatment. Prior ED admissions. Other possibilities: croup, allergic reaction, foreign body ingestion, etc.

➕—Improve oxygenation and ventilation; reduce distress and work of breathing, POC. Monitor: BP, HR, RR, ECG, SpO$_2$, ETCO$_2$, serial auscultation of chest. Consider O$_2$, nebulized bronchodilators; Epinephrine (1:1,000) 0.01 mg/kg (0.01 mL/kg) (maximum dose: 0.3–0.5 mg), administered subcutaneously. For severe asthma, consider Epinephrine (1:10,000) 0.01 mg/kg (0.1 mL/kg) (maximum dose: 0.3 mg), slow IV push every 5 minutes as needed; Solu-Medrol 2 mg/kg IV; Magnesium Sulfate.

Cautions—Remember: "All that wheezes is not asthma."

Croup

HX—Cold or flu that develops into a **"barking cough"** at night. Relatively slow onset. Low fever.

➕—**Cool, moist air; contact OLMC regarding transport. Consider nebulized epi if age >6 months.**

Cautions—Do not examine the upper airway.

Epiglottitis

HX—Cold or flu that develops into a high fever at night. **Drooling, difficulty swallowing**, relatively rapid onset. Inspiratory stidor may be present in severe cases.

➕—**Cool, moist air. If airway is completely obstructed, ventilate with BVM and O$_2$.**

Cautions—Do not examine the upper airway. This may cause total airway obstruction.

Notes

Metric Conversions

TEMPERATURE		WEIGHT		OTHER
°F	**°C**	**Lbs**	**Kg**	**Volume**
106	41.1	396	180	1 tsp = 5 mL
105	40.6	374	170	1 tbsp = 15 mL
104	40	352	160	1 fl. oz. = 30 mL
103	39.4	330	150	1 qt = 946 mL
102	38.9	308	140	
101	38.3	286	130	**Length**
100	37.8	264	120	3/8" = 1 cm
99	37.2	242	110	1" = 2.54 cm
98.6	**37**	**220**	**100**	39.4" = 1 meter
98	36.7	209	95	
97	36.1	198	90	**Weight**
96	35.6	187	85	1/150 gr = 0.4 mg
95	35	176	80	1/100 gr = 0.6 mg
94	34.4	165	75	1/65 gr = 1 mg
93	33.9	154	70	1 gr = 65 mg
92	33.3	143	65	15 gr = 1 gm
91	32.8	132	60	1 gm = 1,000 mg
90	32.2	121	55	1 mg = 1,000 mcg
89	31.7	110	50	1 oz. = 28 gm
88	31.1	99	45	1 lb = 454 gm
87	30.6	88	40	2.2 lbs = 1 kg
86	30	77	35	
85	29.4	66	30	**Pressure**
84	28.9	55	25	1 mm Hg =
83	28.3	44	20	1.36 cm H_2O
82	27.8	33	15	
81	27.2	22	10	
80	26.7	15	7	**"3:00AM Rule"**
75	23.8	11	5	To convert lbs→kg,
70	21.1	7.5	3.5	divide lbs. by 2
65	18.3	5	2.3	and subtract 10%.
32	0	3	1.4	

Common Lab Values

(Adult—blood, plasma, or serum)

NOTE: Normal values may vary, depending on the lab or methods used.

Acetone: 0.3–2 mg%

Alcohol (ETOH): 0 mg%; coma: ≥400–500 mg%

Ammonia: 40–70 mcg

Amylase: 30–110 U/mL, or 80–180 Somogyi units/100 mL

Aspartate aminotransferase (AST): 5–35 U/L

Bicarbonate (HCO_3^-): 23–29 mEq/L

Bilirubin, direct: 0.1–0.4 mg% (total: 0.3–1.1 mg%)

C-reactive protein: <0.8 mg%

Calcium: 4.5–5.5 mEq/L (8.5–11 mg%)

Chloride: 98–109 mEq/L

CO (carbon monoxide): symptoms at ≥10% saturation

CO_2 content: 24–30 mEq/L; infants: 20–26 mEq/L

Creatine kinase MB (CK-MB): 0–5 U/L

Creatinine: 0.7–1.4 mg%

Fibrinogen (plasma): 200–400 mg%

Glucose (fasting): 65–110 mg%; diuresis: ≥180 mg%

Hematocrit: Male: 47% (40–50%): Female: 42% (37–47%)

Hemoglobin (Hgb): Male: 14–18 gm%; Female: 12–16 gm%; Child: 12–14 gm%; Newborn: 15–25 gm%

Iron: 75–175 γ% (less in females)

Lactic dehydrogenase (LDH): 132–240 U/L

Lead: <25 mcg%

Lithium: 0.5–1.5 mEq/L (toxicity ≥2 mEq/L)

Magnesium: 1.5–2.5 mEq/L (1.8–3 mg%)

Myoglobin: 10–65 (95 males)

pCO_2 (arterial): 35–45 torr; Newborn: 35–40 torr

pH (arterial): 7.35–7.45 (mean: 7.40)

pO_2 (arterial): 75–100 torr (avg-room air at sea level)

Platelets: 150,000–400,000/cu mm

Potassium: 3.5–5.0 mEq/L (14–20 mg%)

Protein: total = 6–8.4 gm%

Salicylate: toxicity ≥30 mg%

Sodium: 136–147 mEq/L (313–334 mg%)

Troponin I: <0.1 ng/mL

Urea nitrogen (BUN): 6–23 mg%

Urine (specific gravity): 1.003–1.030

Spanish Translations

(In Spanish, "h" is silent; "ll" is pronounced like "y" [yell]; "j" like "h" [ham]; "qu" like "k" [keep]; and "ñ" like "nya" [canyon]. An accented vowel [á, ó, etc.] simply indicates the syllable that must be stressed when pronouncing the word.)

History and Examination

I am a paramedic (firefighter; nurse; doctor).	Soy paramédico (bombero; enfermera/enfermero; médico).
I speak a little Spanish.	Hablo un poco de español.
Is there someone here that speaks English?	¿Alguien habla inglés?
What is your name?	¿Cómo se llama usted?
I don't understand.	No entiendo.
Can you speak more slowly please?	¿Puede hablar más despacio, por favor?
Wake up sir/madam.	Despierte, señor/señora.
Sit up.	Siéntese.
Listen.	Escúcheme.
How are you?	¿Cómo se siente?
Do you have neck or back pain?	¿Le duele el cuello o la espalda?
Were you unconscious?	¿Estuvo inconsciente?
Move your fingers and toes.	Mueva los dedos de las manos y los pies.
What day is today?	¿Qué día es hoy?
Where is this?	¿Dónde estámos?
Where are you?	¿Dónde está usted?
What is your telephone number? ...address?	¿Cuál es su número de teléfono? ...domicilio?
When were you born?	¿Cuándo nació?
Sit here please.	Siéntese aquí, por favor.
Lie down please.	Acuéstese, por favor.

122

Trouble breathing?	¿Dificultad para respirar?
Weakness?	¿Debilidad?
Where?	¿Dónde?
Show me where it hurts with your hand.	Muéstreme con su mano dónde le duele.
Does the pain increase when you breathe?	¿El dolor aumenta al respirar?
Breathe deeply through your mouth.	Respire profundo por la boca.
Breathe slowly.	Respire lentamente.
Have you been drinking?	¿Ha estado tomando alcohol?
Have you taken any drugs?	¿Ha tomado alguna droga?
Do you have chest pain?	¿Tiene dolor en el pecho?
...heart problems?	...problemas del corazón?
...diabetes?	...diabetes?
...asthma?	...asma?
...allergies?	...alergias?
When were you born?	¿Cuándo nació?
Have you had this pain before?	¿Ha tenido el mismo dolor en otras ocasiones?
How long ago?	¿Hace cúanto tiempo?
Are you sick to your stomach?	¿Tiene náuseas o asco?
Are you pregnant?	¿Está embarazada?
Do you need to vomit?	¿Quiere vomitar?
You will be okay.	Todo saldrá bien.
It is not serious.	No es grave.
It is serious.	Es grave.

Treatment

Please don't move	Por favor, no se mueva.
What's the matter?	¿Qué pasa?
Do you want to go to the hospital?	¿Quieres ir al hospital?
To which hospital?	¿A cuál hospital?
You must go to the hospital.	Tiene que ir al hospital.
We're going to take you to the hospital.	Vamos a llevarte al hospital.
We are going to give you oxygen.	Vamos a darle oxígeno.
We are going to apply a C-collar.	Vamos a ponerle un collarín.
We are going to give you an IV.	Vamos a ponerle un suero.

Miscellaneous

Thank you.	Gracias.	head	la cabeza
Excuse me.	Disculpe.	heart	el corazón
Hello.	Hola.	to help	ayudar
Goodbye.	Adiós.	hip	la cadera
Yes.	Sí.	hypertension	hipertensión/ presión alta
No.	No.	leg	la pierna
abdomen	el abdomen	lungs	los pulmones
ankle	el tobillo	meds	medicinas
arm	el brazo	mouth	la boca
back	la espalda	neck	el cuello
bone	el hueso	penis	el pene
cancer	cáncer	stretcher	la camilla
chest	el pecho	stroke	ataque cerebral
drugs	drogas	throat	la garganta
ear	el oído	vagina	la vagina
eye	el ojo	wrist	la muñeca
foot	el pie		
fracture	una fractura		
hand	la mano		

Prescription Drugs

[UPPER CASE = Brand name; lower case = generic name]
(See last pages for abbreviations.)

A

ABILIFY (aripiprazole): antipsychotic, Rx: schizophrenia
Acarbose (PRECOSE): oral hypoglycemic, Rx: diabetes
ACCOLATE (zafirlukast): bronchospasm inhibitor, Rx: asthma
ACCUNEB (albuterol): beta$_2$ agonist bronchodilator, Rx: asthma, COPD
ACCUPRIL (quinapril): ACE inhibitor, Rx: HTN, CHF
ACCURETIC (quinapril/HCTZ): ACE inhibitor/diuretic, Rx: HTN
Acebutolol (SECTRAL): beta blocker, Rx: HTN, angina, dysrhythmias
ACEON (perindopril): ACE inhibitor, Rx: HTN, CAD
Acetaminophen (TYLENOL): non-narcotic analgesic
Acetazolamide (DIAMOX): diuretic/anticonvulsant, Rx: glaucoma, edema in CHF, epilepsy, mountain sickness
Acetylcysteine (MUCOMYST, ACETADOTE): mucolytic, antidote, Rx: respiratory diseases, acetaminophen overdose, radiocontrast induced nephropathy
ACIPHEX (rabeprazole): inhibits gastric acid secretion, Rx: ulcers, GERD, Zollinger-Ellison syndrome
ACTICIN (permethrin): scabicide, Rx: scabies
ACTIFED (triprolidine/pseudoephedrine): antihistamine/decongestant, Rx: allergies, hay fever, cold
ACTIGALL (ursodiol): bile acid, Rx: gallstones
ACTIQ (fentanyl): oral transmucosal narcotic analgesic, Rx: chronic cancer pain
ACTIVELLA (norethindrone and estradiol): oral and transdermal patch, Rx: menopause
ACTONEL (risedronate): reduces bone loss, Rx: osteoporosis, Paget's disease
ACTOS (pioglitazone): oral hypoglycemic, Rx: diabetes
ACULAR (ketorolac): NSAID analgesic, Rx: ocular itching or pain

Acyclovir (ZOVIRAX): antiviral, Rx: herpes, shingles, chicken pox

ADALAT, ADALAT CC (nifedipine): calcium channel blocker, Rx: angina, HTN

ADDERALL (amphetamines): CNS stimulant, Rx: ADHD, narcolepsy

ADIPEX-P (phentermine hydrochloride): adjunct in exogenous obesity, Rx: obesity

ADRENALIN (epinephrine): bronchodilator, vasopressor, Rx: asthma, life-threatening allergic reactions

ADVAIR DISKUS (fluticasone/salmeterol): inhaled steroid/beta$_2$ bronchodilator, Rx: asthma, COPD

ADVICOR (niacin/lovastatin): antihyperlipidemic, Rx: hypercholesterolemia

ADVIL (ibuprofen): NSAID analgesic, Rx: pain

AEROBID, AEROBID M (flunisolide): inhaled steroid, Rx: asthma, bronchitis

AGGRENOX (aspirin/dipyridamole): antiplatelet agents, Rx: to reduce the risk of stroke

AGRYLIN (anagrelide): reduces platelet count, Rx: thrombocythemia, myeloproliferative disorders

ALAMAST (pemirolast): ophthalmic anti-inflammatory, Rx: allergic conjunctivitis

Albendazole (ALBENZA): anthelmintic, Rx: tapeworm

ALBENZA (albendazole): anthelmintic, Rx: tapeworm

Albuterol (PROVENTIL): beta$_2$ agonist bronchodilator, Rx: asthma, COPD

ALDACTAZIDE (HCTZ/spironolactone): diuretics, Rx: HTN, fluid retention

ALDACTONE (spironolactone): potassium-sparing diuretic, Rx: CHF, ESLD, HTN

ALDOMET (methyldopa): centrally acting antihypertensive, Rx: HTN

Alendronate (FOSOMAX): reduces bone loss, Rx: osteoporosis, Paget's disease

ALESSE (levonorgestrel and ethinyl estradiol): prevention of pregnancy, Rx: oral contraceptive

ALEVE (naproxen): NSAID analgesic, Rx: pain

ALLEGRA (fexofenadine): antihistamine, Rx: allergies

Allopurinol (ZYLOPRIM): xanthine oxidase inhibitor, Rx: gout

ALORA (estradiol): estrogen derivative, Rx: menopause

Alosetron (LOTRONEX): antidiarrheal, Rx: irritable bowel

ALPHAGAN P OPTH (brimonidine): alpha adrenergic agonist, Rx: glaucoma, ocular hypertension

Alprazolam (XANAX): benzodiazepine, Rx: anxiety disorders, panic attacks

ALTACE (ramipril): ACE inhibitor, Rx: HTN, CHF post MI

ALUPENT (metaproterenol): beta$_2$ agonist bronchodilator, Rx: asthma, bronchitis, COPD

Amantadine (SYMMETREL): antiviral, antiparkinsonian, Rx: influenza A, Parkinson's disease

AMARYL (glimepiride): oral hypoglycemic, Rx: diabetes mellitus

AMBIEN (zolpidem): sedative, Rx: insomnia

AMBISOME (amphotericin B lipid-based): antifungal, Rx: fungal infections

AMERGE (naratriptan): selective serotonin receptor agonist, Rx: acute migraine headache

AMEVIVE (B 9273, BG 9273, fusion protein-human): Rx: psoriasis

Amikacin (AMIKIN): aminoglycoside antibiotic, Rx: bacterial infections

AMIKIN (amikacin): aminoglycoside antibiotic, Rx: bacterial infections

Amiloride (MIDAMOR): diuretic, Rx: HTN, fluid retention

Amiloride/HCTZ (MODURETIC): diuretics, Rx: HTN, fluid retention

Aminophylline: bronchodilator, Rx: COPD, asthma, bronchitis

Aminosalicylic Acid (PASER): antibacterial, Rx: tuberculosis

Amiodarone (CORDARONE, PACERONE): antiarrhythmic, Rx: dysrhythmias

Amitriptyline: a tricyclic antidepressant, Rx: depression, neuropathic pain

AMITIZA (lubiprostone): intestinal stimulant, Rx: chronic idiopathic constipation

Amlodipine (LOTREL): calcium channel blocker, Rx: HTN, angina

Amoxapine (ASENDIN): tricyclic antidepressant

Amoxicillin (AMOXIL): penicillin class antibiotic

AMOXIL (amoxicillin): penicillin class antibiotic

Amoxicillin/Clavulanate (Augmentin): penicillin class antibiotic

Amphetamine (ADDERALL): stimulant, Rx: ADHD

Amphotericin B (FUNGIZONE): antifungal agent, Rx: fungal infections

Ampicillin: penicillin class antibiotic

Anagrelide (Agrylin): reduces platelet count, Rx: thrombocythemia, myeloprol

ANAFRANIL (clomipramine): tricyclic antidepressant, Rx: obsessive-compulsive disorder

ANAPROX, ANAPROX DS (naproxen): NSAID analgesic,
Rx: arthritis, pain

Anastrozole (ARIMIDEX): estrogen inhibitor, antineoplastic,
Rx: breast cancer

ANCOBON (flucytosine): antifungal agent, Rx: fungal infections

ANDRODERM (testosterone): androgen replacement therapy,
Rx: hypogonadism

ANTABUSE (disulfiram): alcohol-abuse deterrent, Rx: alcohol abuse

ANTIVERT (meclizine): antiemetic, Rx: motion sickness

ANUSOL HC (hydrocortisone): relief of inflammation,
Rx: corticosteroid anti-inflammatory

ANZEMET (dolasetron): antiemetic, Rx: nausea and vomiting
caused by chemotherapy, anesthesia, or surgery

APAP (acetaminophen): a non-narcotic analgesic, Rx: mild to
moderate pain

APRI (desogestrel and ethinyl): prevention of pregnancy,
Rx: contraceptive

AQUAMEPHYTON (vitamin K): Rx: bleeding disorder of newborn

ARALEN (chloroquine): antimalarial agent, Rx: malaria

ARANESP (darbepoetin): erythropoiesis stimulating agent,
Rx: anemia

ARAVA (leflunomide): immunomodulator agent, Rx: rheumatoid
arthritis

ARICEPT (donepezil): cholinergic enhancer, Rx: dementia
associated with Alzheimer's

ARIMIDEX (anastrozole): estrogen inhibitor, Rx: breast cancer

ARISTOCORT (triamcinolone): corticosteroid, Rx: arthritis, severe
allergies, asthma

ARIXTRA (fondaparinux): anticoagulant, Rx: treatment and
prophylaxis for DVT/PE

ARMOUR THYROID: thyroid hormone, Rx: hypothyroidism

AROMASIN (exemestane): decreases estrogen production,
Rx: breast cancer

ARTHROTEC (diclofenac/misoprostol): NSAID analgesic, antiulcer,
Rx: arthritis

Ascorbic Acid (vitamin C): prevention of scurvy, Rx: urinary
acidification

Aspirin (acetylsalicylic acid, ASA): NSAID analgesic, Rx: pain

ASACOL (mesalamine): anti-inflammatory agent, Rx: colitis

ASTELIN (azelastine): antihistamine, Rx: allergic rhinitis

ASTRAMORPH PF (morphine): narcotic analgesic, Rx: pain
ATACAND (candesartan): ACE inhibitor, Rx: HTN, CHF
ATARAX (hydroxyzine): antihistamine, Rx: itching caused by allergies, motion sickness, alcohol withdrawal
Atenolol (TENORMIN): beta blocker, Rx: HTN, angina, acute MI
Atenolol/Chlorthalidone (TENORETIC): beta blocker/diuretic, Rx: HTN
ATIVAN (lorazepam): benzodiazepine hypnotic, Rx: anxiety
Atovaquone (MEPRON): antiprotozoal, Rx: prophylaxis and treatment for P. carinii pneumonia
ATRIPLA (tenofovir, emtricitabine, efavirenz): antiretrovirals, Rx: HIV/AIDS
ATROVENT (ipratropium): inhaled anticholinergic bronchodilator, Rx: COPD
AUGMENTIN (amoxicillin, clavulanate potassium): penicillin class antibiotic, Rx: bacterial infection
AURALGAN (benzocaine/antipyrine): otic analgesic, Rx: acute otitis media
AVALIDE (irbesartan/hydrochlorothiazide): angiotensin receptor blocker/diuretic, Rx: HTN
AVANDAMET (rosiglitazone/metformin): oral hypoglycemic combination, Rx: diabetes
AVANDIA (rosiglitazone): oral hypoglycemic, Rx: diabetes
AVAPRO (irbesartan): angiotensin receptor blocker, Rx: HTN, diabetic nephropathy
AVELOX (moxifloxacin): fluoroquinolone antibiotic, Rx: bronchitis, pneumonia
AVINZA (morphine ER): narcotic analgesic, Rx: severe pain
AVODART (dutasteride): androgen inhibitor, Rx: benign prostatic hypertrophy
AVONEX (interferon): immunomodulator, Rx: multiple sclerosis
AXERT (almotriptan): selective serotonin receptor agonist, Rx: migraine headaches
AXID (nizatidine): histamine-2 antagonist, inhibits gastric acid secretion, Rx: ulcers
AYGESTIN (norethindrone): hormone, Rx: amenorrhea, endometriosis
AZACTAM (aztreonam): monobactam antibiotic, Rx: bacterial infections
Azathioprine (IMURAN): immunosuppressant, Rx: organ transplants, lupus, rheumatoid arthritis

Azelastine (OPTIVAR): antihistamine, Rx: hayfever, allergies

AZILECT (rasagiline): MAO-B inhibitor, slows metabolism of dopamine, Rx: Parkinson's disease

Azithromycin (ZITHROMAX): macrolide antibiotic, Rx: bacterial infection

AZMACORT (triamcinolone): inhaled corticosteroid, Rx: asthma

AZOPT OPTH (brinzolamide): carbonic anhydrase inhibitor, Rx: glaucoma, ocular hypertension

AZT (zidovudine): antiretroviral agent, Rx: HIV

Aztreonam (AZACTAM): monobactam antibiotic, Rx: bacterial infections

AZULFIDINE-EN (sulfasalazine): anti-inflammatory, Rx: ulcerative colitis, arthritis

B

B&O SUP (belladonna/opium): antispasmodic/analgesic, Rx: ureteral spasm pain

Baclofen: muscle relaxant, Rx: spasm in Ms, spinal cord disease.

Balsalazide (COLAZAL): anti-inflammatory, Rx: ulcerative colitis

BARACLUDE (entecavir): antiretroviral agent, reverse transcriptase inhibitor (nucleoside), Rx: hepatitis B

Beclomethasone (QVAR): inhaled corticosteroid, Rx: asthma

BECONASE AQ (beclomethasone): nasal steroid, Rx: allergies

Belladonna alkaloids with Phenobarbital (DONNATAL): antispasmodic, Rx: irritable bowel

BENADRYL (diphenhydramine): histamine H_1 antagonist, Rx: antihistamine

Benazepril (LOTENSIN): ACE inhibitor, Rx: HTN

Benazepril/HCTZ (LOTENSIN HCT): ACE inhibitor/diuretic, Rx: HTN

BENICAR (olmesartan): angiotensin II receptor antagonist, Rx: HTN

BENTYL (dicyclomine): anticholinergic, Rx: irritable bowel

Benzonatate (TESSALON): antitussive, Rx: cough

Benzoyl Peroxide (PANOXYL): antibacterial, Rx: acne

Benzphetamine (DIDREX): amphetamine, Rx: obesity

Benztropine (COGENTIN): anticholinergic, Rx: Parkinson's disease, extrapyramidal disorders

BETAGAN OPTH (levobunolol): beta blocker, lowers intraocular pressure, Rx: glaucoma

Betamethasone (CELESTONE): corticosteroid anti-inflammatory

BETAPACE (sotalol): antiarrhythmic, Rx: dysrhythmias

BETASERON (interferon): immunomodulator, Rx: Multiple Sclerosis
Betaxolol (KERLONE): beta blocker, Rx: HTN
Bethanechol (URECHOLINE): urinary cholinergic, Rx: urinary retention
BETOPTIC (betaxolol): ophthalmic beta blocker, Rx: glaucoma
BIAXIN (clarithromycin): macrolide antibiotic, Rx: bacterial infections
BICILLIN (penicillin): penicillin antibiotic, Rx: bacterial infections
BIDIL (hydralazine/isosorbide dinitrate): vasodilators, Rx: heart failure
Bisacodyl (DULCOLAX): laxative, Rx: constipation
Bismuth (PEPTO-BISMOL): gastrointestinal, Rx: indigestion, diarrhea
Bisoprolol (Zebeta): beta blocker, Rx: HTN
Bisoprolol/HCTZ (ZIAC): beta blocker/diuretic, Rx: HTN
Bleomycin: antineoplastic, Rx: lymphomas, pleural effusions
BLEPHAMIDE (sulfacetamide/prednisolone): antibiotic/steroid, Rx: eye infection/inflammation
BONIVA (ibandronate): osteoclast inhibitor, Rx: osteoporosis
BRETHINE (terbutaline): beta$_2$ agonist, Rx: COPD, asthma
BREVICON: oral contraceptive
Brimonidine (ALPHAGAN): alpha-2 agonist, Rx: glaucoma, ocular hypertension
Brinzolamide (AZOPT OPHTHALMIC): alpha adrenergic agonist, Rx: glaucoma, ocular hypertension
Bromocriptine (PARLODEL): dopamine agonist, Rx: Parkinson's disease, hyperprolactinemia, acromegaly
Brompheniramine (BROMFED): antihistamine, Rx: allergies
BROVANA (arformoterol): beta$_2$ adenergic agonist, long acting, Rx: COPD
Budesonide (RHINOCORT, PULMICORT): nasal, inhaled corticosteroid, Rx: allergic rhinitis, asthma
Bumetanide (BUMEX): diuretic, Rx: edema, CHF
BUPAP (butalbital, acetaminophen): sedative analgesic, Rx: tension headache
Buprenorphine: opioid partial agonist-antagonist, Rx: opioid dependence
Bupropion (WELLBUTRIN, ZYBAN): antidepressant, Rx: depression, smoking cessation
Buspirone (BUSPAR): antianxiety agent, Rx: anxiety disorders
Busulfan (MYLERAN): anticancer agent, Rx: chronic myelogenous leukemia
Butalbital/Acetaminophen/Caffeine (FIORICET/ESGIC): sedative analgesic, Rx: tension headache

Butalbital/Aspirin/Caffeine (FIORINAL): sedative analgesic, Rx: tension headache

Butenafine (MENTAX): antifungal, Rx: fungal infections

Butoconazole (MYCELEX-3): antifungal, Rx: vaginal candidiasis

Butorphanol (STADOL): opioid analgesic, Rx: pain

BYETTA (exenatide): enhances insulin secretion, Rx: diabetes (type 2)

BYSTOLIC (nebivolol hydrochloride): beta blocker, Rx: hypertension

C

CADUET (amlodipine/atorvastatin): calcium channel blocker/antihyperlipidemic

CAFERGOT (ergotamine/caffeine): vasoconstrictors, Rx: migraine/tension headache

CALAN, CALAN SR (verapamil): calcium channel blocker, Rx: angina, hypertension, prophylaxis headache, dysrhythmias

CALCIFEROL (ergocalciferol): vitamin D, Rx: hypocalcemia, hypoparathyroidism, rickets, osteodystrophy

CALCIJEX (calcitriol): vitamin D supplement, Rx: hypocalcemia in renal disease, hypoparathyroidism, bone disease

Calcipotriene (DOVONEX): vitamin D agonist, Rx: psoriasis

Calcitonin-Salmon (MIACALCIN): bone resorption inhibitor hormone, Rx: hypercalcemia, Paget's disease, osteoporosis

Calcitriol (CALCIJEX, ROCALTROL): vitamin D supplement, Rx: hypocalcemia in renal disease, hypoparathyroidism, bone disease

CALDOLOR (ibuprofen): injectable NSAID analgesic, Rx: pain, fever

CAMILA (norethindrone): contraceptive, Rx: amenorrhea, endometriosis, pregnancy prevention

CAMPRAL (acamprosate): reduces alcohol withdrawal symptoms, Rx: alcohol dependence

CANASA (mesalamine): 5-aminosalicylic acid derivative, Rx: ulcerative colitis

Candesartan Cilexetil (ATACAND): ACE inhibitor, Rx: HTN, CHF

CAPITAL with Codeine (APAP/codeine): narcotic analgesic, Rx: mild to moderate pain

CAPOTEN (captopril): ACE inhibitor, Rx: CHF, HTN, diabetic nephropathy

Captopril (CAPOTEN): ACE inhibitor, Rx: HTN, CHF, diabetic nephropathy

CARAFATE (sucralfate): gastrointestinal agent, Rx: duodenal ulcer

Carbamazepine (CARBATROL, TEGRETOL): anticonvulsant, Rx: seizures, trigeminal neuralgia, bipolar disorder
CARBATROL (carbamazepine): anticonvulsant, Rx: seizures, trigeminal neuralgia, bipolar disorder
Carbidopa/Levodopa (SINEMET, PARCOPA): dopamine precursors, Rx: Parkinson's disease
CARDIZEM (diltiazem): antiarrhythmic agent, calcium channel blocker, Rx: angina, hypertension, atrial fibrillation, atrial flutter, paroxysmal supraventricular tachycardia
CARDURA (doxazosin): alpha blocker, Rx: HTN, benign prostatic hypertrophy
CAREFGOT (ergotamine/caffeine): vasoconstrictors, Rx: migraine/tension headache
Carisoprodol (SOMA): muscle relaxant, Rx: musculoskeletal pain
CARTIA XT (diltiazem): antiarrhythmic agent, calcium channel blocker, Rx: angina, hypertension, atrial fibrillation, atrial flutter, paroxysmal supraventricular tachycardia
Carvedilol (COREG): beta and alpha blocker, Rx: angina, heart failure, HTN
CASODEX (bicalutamide): antiandrogen, Rx: prostate cancer
Caspofungin (CANCIDAS): antifungal agent, Rx: fungal infection
CATAPRES, CATAPRES TTS (clonidine): centrally acting alpha agonist, Rx: HTN
CAUDET (amlodipine/atorvastatin): calcium blocker/lipid lowering agent, Rx: HTN and high cholesterol
CECLOR (cefaclor): cephalosporin antibiotic, Rx: bacterial infections
CEDAX (ceftibuten): cephalosporin antibiotic, Rx: bacterial infections
Cefaclor (CECLOR): cephalosporin antibiotic, Rx: bacterial infections
Cefadroxil (DURICEF): cephalosporin antibiotic, Rx: bacterial infections
Cefazolin (ANCEF): cephalosporin antibiotic, Rx: bacterial infections
Cefdinir (OMNICEF): cephalosporin antibiotic, Rx: bacterial infections
Cefepime (MAXIPIME): cephalosporin antibiotic, Rx: bacterial infections
Cefixime (SUPRAX): cephalosporin antibiotic, Rx: bacterial infections
CEFIZOX (ceftizoxime): cephalosporin antibiotic, Rx: bacterial infections
Cefotaxime (CLAFORAN): cephalosporin antibiotic, Rx: bacterial infections
Cefotetan (CEFOTAN): cephalosporin antibiotic, Rx: bacterial infections

Cefoxitin (MEFOXIN): cephalosporin antibiotic, Rx: bacterial infections

Cefpodoxime (VANTIN): cephalosporin antibiotic, Rx: bacterial infections

Cefprozil (CEFZIL): cephalosporin antibiotic, Rx: bacterial infections

Ceftazidime (FORTAZ): cephalosporin antibiotic, Rx: bacterial infections

Ceftibuten (CEDAX): cephalosporin antibiotic, Rx: bacterial infections

CEFTIN (cefuroxime): cephalosporin antibiotic, Rx: bacterial infections

Ceftizoxime (CEFIZOX): cephalosporin antibiotic, Rx: bacterial infections

Ceftriaxone (ROCEPHIN): cephalosporin antibiotic, Rx: bacterial infections

Cefuroxime (CEFTIN): cephalosporin antibiotic, Rx: bacterial infections

CEFZIL (cefprozil): cephalosporin antibiotic, Rx: bacterial infections

CELEBREX (celecoxib): NSAID, Rx: arthritis, acute pain

CELEXA (citalopram): SSRI, Rx: depression

CELLCEPT (mycophenolate): immunosuppressant, Rx: organ transplants

CELONTIN (methsuximide): anticonvulsant, Rx: absence seizure

Cephalexin (KEFLEX): cephalosporin antibiotic, Rx: bacterial infections

CEREBYX (fosphenytoin): anticonvulsant, Rx: epilepsy

Cetirizine (ZYRTEC): antihistamine, Rx: allergic rhinitis, urticaria

Cevimeline (EVOXAC): cholinergic, Rx: dry mouth from Sjogren's syndrome

CHANTIX (varenicline): nicotine receptor stimulator, Rx: smoking cessation

Chloral Hydrate: sedative/hypnotic, Rx: insomnia, pain, alcohol withdrawal

Chlorambucil (LEUKERAN): alkylating agent, Rx: leukemia, lymphomas, Hodgkin's disease

Chlordiazepoxide (LIBRIUM): benzodiazepine, Rx: anxiety, agitation from alcohol withdrawal

Chlorhexidine (PERIDEX): antimicrobial rinse, Rx: gingivitis

Chloroquine (ARALEN): antimalarial, amebicidal agent, Rx: malaria

Chlorothiazide (DIURIL): diuretic, Rx: fluid retention in CHF, renal failure, HTN

Chlorpheniramine (CHLOR-TRIMETON): antihistamine, Rx: colds, allergies
Chlorpromazine (THORAZINE): antipsychotic, Rx: schizophrenia
Chlorthalidone (HYGROTON): diuretic, Rx: fluid retention in CHF, renal failure, HTN
Chlorzoxazone (PARAFON FORTE): skeletal muscle relaxant
Cholestyramine (QUESTRAN): bile acid sequestrant, Rx: antihyperlipidemic
CIALIS (tadalafil): vasodialator, Rx: male erectile dysfunction
Ciclopirox (LOPROX): antifungal, Rx: ringworm, candida
Cidofovir (VISTIDE): antiviral, Rx: cytomegalovirus in AIDS
Cilostazol (PLETAL): vasodilator, platelet inhibitor, Rx: leg cramps
Cimetidine (TAGAMET): histamine-2 blocker, inhibits gastric acid secretion, Rx: ulcers
CIPRO (ciprofloxacin): fluoroquinolone antibiotic, Rx: bacterial infections
CIPRODEX (ciprofloxacin/dexamethasone): antibiotic/steroid, Rx: ear infection
Ciprofloxacin (CIPRO): fluoroquinolone antibiotic, Rx: bacterial infections
Cisplatin (PLATINOL AQ): antineoplastic, Rx: ovarian/testicular/bladder cancer
Citalopram (CELEXA): SSRI, Rx: depression
Cladribine (LEUSTATIN): antineoplastic, Rx: leukemia
CLAFORAN (cefotaxime): cephalosporin antibiotic, Rx: bacterial infections
CLARINEX (desloratadine): antihistamine, Rx: urticaria, allergies
Clarithromycin (BIAXIN): macrolide antibiotic, Rx: bacterial infections
CLEOCIN (clindamycin tropical): antibiotic, Rx: acne, Gardnerella vaginalis
CLEVIPREX (clevidipine): calcium channel blocker, Rx: HTN
CLIMARA (estradiol): transdermal estrogen, Rx: symptoms of menopause
Clindamycin (CLEOCIN): antibiotic, Rx: bacterial infections
CLINORIL (sulindac): NSAID analgesic, Rx: arthritis, acute pain
Clomipramine (ANAFRANIL): tricyclic compound, Rx: obsessive-compulsive disorder
Clonazepam (KLONOPIN): anticonvulsant, Rx: seizures, panic disorders

Clonidine (CATAPRES): centrally acting alpha agonist, Rx: HTN

Clopidogrel (PLAVIX): antiplatelet, Rx: ACS, AMI, stroke

Clorazepate (TRANXENE): benzodiazepine, Rx: anxiety/seizure

Clotrimazole (MYCELEX, LOTRIMIN AF): antifungal, Rx: fungal infection

Clozapine (CLOZARIL): antipsychotic, Rx: schizophrenia

CLOZARIL (clozapine): antipsychotic, Rx: schizophrenia

Codeine: narcotic analgesic/antitussive

COGENTIN (benztropine): anticholinergic, Rx: Parkinson's disease, extrapyramidal disorders

COGNEX (tacrine): cholinesterase inhibitor, Rx: Alzheimer's disease

COLACE (docusate): stool softener, Rx: constipation

COLAZAL (balsalazide): anti-inflammatory, Rx: ulcerative colitis

Colchicine: anti-inflammatory, Rx: gout

Colesevelam (WELCHOL): bile acid sequestrant, Rx: hyperlipidemia

COLESTID (colestipol): bile acid sequestrant, Rx: hyperlipidemia

Colestipol (COLESTID): bile acid sequestrant, Rx: hyperlipidemia

Colistimethate (COLY-MYCIN M): antibiotic, Rx: pseudomonas infection

COLY-MYCIN M (colistimethane): antibiotic, Rx: pseudomonas infection

COMBIPATCH (estradiol/norethindrone): estrogens, Rx: menopause symptoms

COMBIVENT (albuterol/ipratropium): bronchodilators, Rx: asthma, COPD

COMBIVIR (lamivudine/zidovudine): antiretrovirals, Rx: HIV

COMPAZINE (prochlorperazine): a phenothiazine antiemetic

COMTAN (entacapone): COMT inhibitor, Rx: Parkinson's disease

CONCERTA (methylphenidate): stimulant, Rx: ADHD, narcolepsy

CONDYLOX (podofilox): antimitotic, Rx: anogenital warts

COPAXONE (glatiramer): immunomodulator, Rx: MS

COPEGUS (ribavirin): antiviral, Rx: hepatitis C

CORDARONE (amiodarone): antiarrhythmic, Rx: dysrhythmias

COREG (carvedilol): beta and alpha blocker, Rx: HTN, CHF, angina

CORGARD (nadolol): beta blocker, Rx: HTN, angina

CORTEF (hydroxycortisone): steroid anti-inflammatory, Rx: arthritis, colitis, allergies, asthma

CORTIC Ear Drops (chloroxylenol/pramoxine/hydrocortisone): antiseptic/antifungal/steroid anti-inflammatory

CORTIFOAM (hydrocortisone): steroid anti-inflammatory, Rx: proctitis, various skin conditions

CORTISOL (hydrocortisone): steroid anti-inflammatory, Rx: arthritis, allergies, asthma

Cortisone: steroid anti-inflammatory, Rx: various skin conditions, allergies, adrenal insufficiency

CORTISPORIN (neomycin/polymyxin/hydrocortisone): antibiotic/steroid anti-inflammatory, Rx: ear, eye, and skin infections

CORVERT (ibutilide): antiarrhythmic, Rx: atrial fibrillation, flutter

COSOPT (timolol/dorzolamide): decreases intraocular pressure, Rx: glaucoma

COUMADIN (warfarin): an anticoagulant, Rx: thrombosis prophylaxis

COVERA HS (verapamil): calcium channel blocker, Rx: HTN, angina, dysrhythmias

COZAAR (losartan): angiotensin receptor blocker, Rx: HTN, diabetic nephropathy

CREON, CREON 5, CREON 10, CREON 20 (pancrelipase): pancreatic enzyme replacement

CRESTOR (rosuvastatin): statin, Rx: hyperlipidemia

CRIXIVAN (indinavir): protease inhibitor antiretroviral, Rx: HIV

Cromolyn (INTAL): anti-inflammatory agent, Rx: asthma prophylaxis, allergies

CRYSELLE (ethinyl estradiol and norgestrel): contraceptive, Rx: prevent pregnancy, "morning after pill"

CUBICIN (daptomycin): lipopeptide antibiotic, Rx: bacterial infections

Cyanocobalamin (vitamin B-12): Rx: anemia

CYCLESSA (ethinyl estradiol and desogestrel): contraceptive, Rx: prevent pregnancy

Cyclobenzaprine (FLEXERIL): skeletal muscle relaxant

CYCLOMYDRIL (cyclopentolate/phenylephrine): production of mydriasis

Cyclosporine (GENGRAF, NEORAL, SANDIMMUNE): immunosuppressant agent, Rx: organ transplants

CYMBALTA (duloxetine): SSRI, Rx: depression, diabetic neuropathy

Cyproheptadine (PERIACTIN): antihistamine

CYTOMEL (liothyronine): thyroid hormone, Rx: hypothyroidism

CYTOTEC (misoprostol): prevents gastric ulcers from NSAIDs

CYTOVENE (ganciclovir): antiviral, Rx: CMV disease

d4T stavudine (ZERIT): antiretroviral, Rx: HIV

DALMANE (flurazepam): benzodiazepine, Rx: insomnia

Danazol: sex hormone, Rx: endometriosis

DANTRIUM (dantrolene): skeletal muscle antispasmodic, Rx: spasm, malignant hyperthermia

Dantrolene (DANTRIUM): skeletal muscle antispasmodic, Rx: spasm, malignant hyperthermia

Dapsone: antibacterial drug, Rx: leprosy, PCP prophylaxis

DARAPRIM (pyrimethamine): antiparasitic, Rx: malaria, toxoplasmosis

DARVOCET-N (propoxyphene/APAP): narcotic analgesic, Rx: mild to moderate pain

DARVON (propoxyphene): narcotic analgesic, Rx: mild to moderate pain

DAYPRO (oxaprozin): NSAID, Rx: arthritis

DDAVP (desmopressin): antidiuretic hormone, Rx: nocturia, diabetes insipidus

DECADRON (dexamethasone): steroid anti-inflammatory, Rx: neoplastic disorders, allergies, GI diseases, endocrine disorders

DECLOMYCIN (demeclocycline): tetracycline antibiotic, Rx: SIADH

Deferoxamine (DESFERAL): iron-chelator, Rx: iron toxicity

Delavirdine (RESCRIPTOR): antiretroviral, Rx: HIV

Deltasone (prednisone): steroid anti-inflammatory

DEMADEX (torsemide): loop diuretic, Rx: HTN, edema in CHF, kidney disease, liver disease

Demeclocycline (DECLOMYCIN): tetracycline antibiotic, Rx: SIADH

DEMEROL (meperidine): opioid analgesic, Rx: moderate to severe pain

DEPACON (divalproex): anticonvulsant, Rx: seizures, bipolar disorder, migraine

DEPAKENE (valproic acid): anticonvulsant, Rx: seizures

DEPAKOTE, DEPAKOTE ER (divalproex): anticonvulsant, antimigraine, Rx: migraine headache, absence seizures

DEPO-MEDROL (methylprednisolone): corticosteroid anti-inflammatory

DEPO-PROVERA (medroxyprogesterone): progesterone, Rx: endometrial or renal cancer

Desipramine (NORPRAMIN): tricyclic antidepressant

Desmopressin (DDAVP): antidiuretic hormone, Rx: nocturia, diabetes insipidus

DESOGEN (etinyl estradiol and desogestrel): contraceptive, Rx: prevent pregnancy

DESOXYN (methamphetamine): amphetamine, Rx: ADHD, obesity

DETROL (tolterodine): urinary bladder antispasmodic, Rx: overactive bladder

Dexamethasone (DECADRON): steroid anti-inflammatory, Rx: neoplastic disorders, allergies, GI diseases, endocrine disorders

DEXEDRINE (dextroamphetamine): amphetamine, Rx: ADHD, narcolepsy

Dextroamphetamine (DEXEDRINE): amphetamine, Rx: ADHD, narcolepsy

Dextroamphetamine/Amphetamine (ADDERALL): amphetamine, Rx: ADHD, narcolepsy

Dextromethorphan (DELSYM, ROBITUSSIN): non-narcotic antitussive

DEXTROSTAT (dextroamphetamine): stimulant, Rx: ADHD, narcolepsy

DIABETA (glyburide): oral hypoglycemic, Rx: diabetes (type 2 only)

DIAMOX (acetazolamide): diuretic/anticonvulsant, Rx: glaucoma, CHF, epilepsy, mountain sickness

Diazepam (VALIUM): anxiolytic, Rx: anxiety, seizure, panic disorder

DIBENZYLINE (phenoxybenzamine): alpha blocker, Rx: pheochromocytoma

Diclofenac (VOLTAREN): NSAID, analgesic, Rx: arthritis, post-operative ocular inflammation

Dicloxacillin: penicillin antibiotic, Rx: bacterial infections

Dicyclomine (BENTYL): anticholinergic, Rx: irritable bowel syndrome

Didanosine, ddi (VIDEX): antiretroviral, Rx: HIV

DIDREX (benzphetamine): amphetamine, Rx: obesity

DIDRONEL (etidronate): bone metabolism regulator, Rx: Paget's disease, total hip replacement

DIFLUCAN (fluconazole): antifungal, Rx: yeast infection

Diflunisal (DOLOBID): NSAID analgesic, Rx: arthritis

DIGITEK (digoxin): cardiac glycoside, Rx: CHF, atrial fibrillation

Digoxin (LANOXIN): cardiac glycoside, Rx: CHF, atrial fibrillation

Dihydroergotamine (D.H.E.): vasoconstrictor, Rx: migraine headache

DILATRATE SR (isosorbide): long-acting nitrate, Rx: angina

DILAUDID (hydromorphone): opioid analgesic, Rx: moderate to severe pain

Diltiazem (CARDIZEM): calcium channel blocker, Rx: angina, HTN, PSVT

Dimenhydrinate (DRAMAMINE): antihistamine, Rx: motion sickness

DIOVAN (valsartan): angiotensin II receptor inhibitor, Rx: HTN, CHF, post MI

DIOVAN HCT (valsartan/HCTZ): angiotensin II receptor inhibitor/diuretic, Rx: HTN

DIPENTUM (olsalazine): anti-inflammatory agent, Rx: ulcerative colitis

Diphenhydramine (BENADRYL): antihistamine, Rx: allergies

Diphenoxylate/Atropine (LOMOTIL): opioid congener, Rx: diarrhea

Dipyridamole (PERSANTINE): antiplatelet, Rx: lowers risk of postoperative thromboembolic complications after heart valve replacement

Disopyramide (NORPACE): antiarrhythmic, Rx: ventricular dysrhythmias

Disulfiram (ANTABUSE): alcohol-abuse deterrent, Rx: alcohol abuse

DITROPAN XL (oxybutynin): anticholinergic/antispasmodic, Rx: urinary frequency, incontinence, dysuria

DIURIL (chlorothiazide): diuretic, Rx: fluid retention in CHF, renal failure, HTN

Divalproex (DEPAKOTE): anticonvulsant, Rx: seizures, bipolar disorder, migraines

Docusate (COLACE): stool softener, Rx: constipation

Dolasetron (ANZEMET): antiemetic, Rx: nausea and vomiting

DOLOBID (diflunisal): NSAID analgesic, Rx: arthritis

DOLOPHINE (methadone): Opioid analgesic, Rx: pain, opiate withdrawal symptoms

Donepezil (ARICEPT): cholinergic, Rx: dementia associated with Alzheimer's disease

DONNATAL (phenobarbital/belladonna alkaloids): barbiturate sedative/antispasmodic, Rx: irritable bowel syndrome

DORIBAX (doripenem): carbapenem antibiotic, Rx: bacterial infections

Dornase Alfa (PULMOZYME): lytic enzyme that dissolves infected lung secretions, Rx: cystic fibrosis

Dorzolamide OPTH (TRUSOPT): decreases intraocular pressure, Rx: glaucoma

Dorzolamide/Timolol OPTH (COSOPT): decreases intraocular pressure, Rx: glaucoma
DOVONEX (calcipotriene): vitamin D analog, Rx: psoriasis
Doxazosin (CARDURA): alpha blocker, Rx: HTN, benign prostatic hypertrophy
Doxepin (SINEQUAN): tricyclic antidepressant, Rx: depression, anxiety
DOXIL (doxorubicin): antineoplastic, Rx: AIDS-related tumors
Doxorubicin (DOXIL): antineoplastic, Rx: AIDS-related tumors, cancer, leukemia
Doxycycline (VIBRAMYCIN): tetracycline antibiotic, Rx: bacterial infections
Doxylamine (UNISOM): antihistamine sedative, Rx: insomnia
DRAMAMINE (dimenhydrinate): antihistamine, Rx: motion sickness
Dronabinol (MARINOL): appetite stimulant, Rx: weight loss in cancer, AIDS
DTIC-DOME (dacarbazine): anticancer agent, Rx: melanomas, Hodgkin's disease
DUONEB (ipratropium/albuterol): bronchodilators, Rx: asthma, COPD
DURAGESIC (fentanyl): transdermal opioid analgesic, Rx: chronic pain
DURAMORPH (morphine): opioid analgesic, Rx: moderate to severe pain
DURATUSS AM/PM PACK GP (guaifenesin/pseudoephedrine): decongestant/expectorant, Rx: colds
DYAZIDE (HCTZ/triamterene): diuretics, Rx: HTN
DYNACIN (minocycline): tetracycline antibiotic, Rx: bacterial infections, acne
DYNACIRC CR (isradipine): calcium channel blocker, Rx: HTN
DYRENIUM (triamterene): potassium-sparing diuretic, Rx: edema in CHF/ESLD/nephrotic syndrome

E

EDECRIN (ethacrynic acid): diuretic, Rx: CHF, pulmonary edema
EES (erythromycin): macrolide antibiotic, Rx: bacterial infection
Efavirenz (SUSTIVA): antiviral, Rx: HIV-I infection
EFFEXOR, EFFEXOR XR (venlafaxine): antidepressant, Rx: depression, anxiety, panic disorder
ELDEPRYL (selegiline): MAO inhibitor, Rx: Parkinson's disease

ELIMITE (permethrin): parasiticide, Rx: scabies, lice

ELOXATIN (oxaliplatin): antineoplastic, Rx: colorectal cancer

ELSPAR (asparginase): antineoplastic, Rx: leukemia, sarcoma

EMCYT (estramustine): antineoplastic, Rx: prostate cancer

EMSAM Patch (selegiline): MAO inhibitor, Rx: depression

EMTRIVA (emtricitabine): antiretroviral, Rx: HIV

ENABLEX (darifenacin): anticholinergic, Rx: overactive bladder

Enalapril, Enalaprilat (VASOTEC): ACE inhibitor, Rx: HTN, CHF

Enalapril/HCTZ (VASORETIC): ACE inhibitor/diuretic, Rx: HTN

ENBREL (etanercept): antirheumatic, Rx: rheumatoid arthritis, psoriasis

ENDOCET (oxycodone/acetaminophen): opioid analgesic, Rx: moderate to severe pain

ENJUVIA (estrogen derivative): synthetic hormone, Rx: menopause symptoms

Entacapone (COMTAN): COMT inhibitor, Rx: Parkinson's disease

ENTEREG (alvimopan): GI opioid antagonist, Rx: postoperative ileus

ENTOCORT EC (budesonide): corticosteroid, Rx: Crohn's disease

Ephedrine: bronchodilator, Rx: asthma, COPD

EPIPEN (epinephrine): bronchodilator/vasoconstrictor, Rx: allergic reaction

EPIVIR, EPIVIR HBV (lamivudine): antiretroviral, Rx: HIV, hepatitis B

Epoetin Alfa (EPOGEN): increases RBC production, Rx: anemia

EPOGEN (epoetin alfa): increases RBC production, Rx: anemia

EPZICOM (abacavir/lamivudine): antiretroviral, Rx: HIV

EQUETRO (carbamazepine): anticonvulsant, Rx: bipolar disorder

ERBITUX (cetuximab): antineoplastic, Rx: colorectal cancer, cancer of head and neck

Ergocalciferol (CALCIFEROL): vitamin D, Rx: hypocalcemia, hypoparathyroidism, rickets, osteodystrophy

ERRIN (norethindrone): contraceptive, progestin, Rx: amenorrhea, prevent pregnancy

ERYC (erythromycin, systemic): antibiotic, Rx: bacterial infections

ERYPED (erythromycin): macrolide antibiotic, Rx: bacterial infection

ERY-TAB (erythromycin): antibiotic, Rx: bacterial infection

Erythromycin (EES): an antibiotic, Rx: bacterial infection

ESGIC, ESGIC-PLUS (APAP/caffeine/butalbital): analgesic/muscle relaxant/antianxiety compound, Rx: headache

ESKALITH, ESKALITH CR (lithium): antipsychotic, Rx: bipolar disorder

Estazolam (PROSOM): sedative/hypnotic, Rx: insomnia

ESTRACE (estradiol): estrogen, Rx: symptoms of menopause

ESTRADERM (estradiol): transdermal estrogen, Rx: symptoms of menopause

Estradiol (CLIMARA): estrogen derivative, systemic, Rx: menopause

ESTRATEST (estrogens/methyltestosterone), Rx: symptoms of menopause

Estropipate (OGEN): estrogens, Rx: symptoms of menopause

ESTROSTEP (ethinyl estradiol and norethindrone): contraceptive, Rx: prevent pregnancy

Ethacrynate (EDECRIN): diuretic, Rx: pulmonary edema, CHF

Ethambutol (MYAMBUTOL): Rx: pulmonary tuberculosis

Ethosuximide (ZARONTIN): anticonvulsant, Rx: absence seizure

Etidronate (DIDRONEL): bone metabolism regulator, Rx: Paget's disease, total hip replacement

Etodolac (LODINE): NSAID analgesic, Rx: arthritis

Etoposide (VEPESID): antineoplastic, Rx: testicular cancer, lung cancer

EULEXIN (flutamide): antiandrogen, Rx: prostate cancer

EVISTA (raloxifene): estrogen modulator, Rx: osteoporosis, breast cancer prevention

EVOXAC (cevimeline): cholinergic, Rx: dry mouth from Sjogren's syndrome

EXELON (rivastigmine): cholinesterase inhibitor, Rx: dementia in Alzheimer's and Parkinson's disease

EXJADE (deferasirox): chelating agent, Rx: iron overload

EXTENDRYL (phenylephrine/methscopolamine/chlorpheniramine): antihistamine/decongestant, Rx: allergies

F

FACTIVE (gemifloxacin): fluoroquinolone antibiotic, Rx: bacterial infections

Famciclovir (FAMVIR): antiviral, Rx: herpes

Famotidine (PEPCID): H-2 blocker, inhibits gastric acid, Rx: ulcers

FAMVIR (famciclovir): antiviral, Rx: herpes

FANAPT (iloperidone): antipsychotic, Rx: schizophrenia

FARESTON (toremifene): antiestrogen, Rx: breast cancer

FAZACLO (clozapine): antipsychotic, Rx: schizophrenia

FELBATOL (felbamate): antiepileptic, Rx: seizures

FELDENE (piroxicam): NSAID analgesic, Rx: arthritis

Felodipine (PLENDIL): calcium channel blocker, Rx: HTN

FEMARA (letrozole): estrogen inhibitor, Rx: breast cancer

FEMHRT (ethinly estradiol and norethindrone): contraceptive, Rx: prevent pregnancy, acne, menopause

Fenofibrate (TRICOR): lipid regulator, Rx: hyperlipidemia

Fenoprofen (NALFON): nonsteroidal anti-inflammatory, Rx: rheumatoid arthritis, pain

Fentanyl (DURAGESIC): opioid analgesic, Rx: moderate to severe pain

FERRLECIT (sodium ferric gluconate): hematinic, Rx: iron deficiency anemia in hemodialysis

Fexofenadine (ALLEGRA): antihistamine, Rx: allergies

FIBERCON (polycarbophil): bulk-producing laxative, Rx: constipation

Finasteride (PROSCAR, PROPECIA): antiandrogen, Rx: hair loss, BPH

FIORICET (butalbital/APAP/caffeine): sedative, analgesic, Rx: tension headache

FIORINAL (butalbital/ASA/caffeine): sedative analgesic, Rx: tension headache

FLAGYL (metronidazole): antibiotic, Rx: bacterial infections

Flecainide (TAMBOCOR): antiarrhythmic, Rx: PSVT, paroxysmal atrial fibrillation

FLEXERIL (cyclobenzaprine): skeletal muscle relaxant

FLOLAN (epoprostenol): vasodilator, platelet inhibitor, Rx: pulmonary hypertension

FLOMAX (tamsulosin): alpha-1 blocker, Rx: BPH

FLONASE (fluticasone): nasal corticosteroid, Rx: allergic rhinitis

FLORINEF (fludrocortisone): mineralocorticoid, Rx: adrenal insufficiency

FLOVENT (fluticasone): inhaled corticosteroid, Rx: asthma

FLOXIN (ofloxacin): fluoroquinolone antibiotic, Rx: bacterial infections

Fluconazole (DIFLUCAN): antifungal, Rx: yeast infection

Flucytosine (ANCOBON): antifungal, Rx: candida, cryptococcus infection

FLUDARA (fludarabine): antineoplastic, Rx: lymphocytic leukemia

Fludarabine (FLUDARA): antineoplastic, Rx: lymphocytic leukemia

Fludrocortisone (FLORINEF): mineralocorticoid, Rx: adrenal insufficiency

FLUMADINE (rimantadine): antiviral, Rx: influenza A virus

144

Flumazenil (ROMAZICON): antidote, Rx: benzodiazepine overdose

Flunisolide (AEROBID): inhaled corticosteroid, Rx: asthma

Flunisolide (NASAREL): nasal corticosteroid, Rx: allergic rhinitis

Fluoxetine (PROZAC): antidepressant, Rx: depression, obsessive-compulsive disorder, bulimia

Fluphenazine: antipsychotic, Rx: schizophrenia

Flurazepam (DALMANE): benzodiazepine, Rx: insomnia

Flurbiprofen (ANSAID): NSAID analgesic, Rx: arthritis

Flutamide (EULEXIN): antiandrogenic, Rx: prostate cancer

Fluvoxamine (LUVOX): SSRI, Rx: obsessive-compulsive disorder, anxiety

FOCALIN (dexmethylphenidate): stimulant, Rx: ADHD

Folic Acid: vitamin coenzyme, Rx: megaloblastic anemia

FORADIL (formoterol): long acting beta$_2$ agonist bronchodilator, Rx: asthma, COPD

FORTAMET (metformin): antidiabetic agent, Rx: diabetes

FORTAZ (ceftazidime): cephalosporin antibiotic, Rx: bacterial infections

FOSAMAX (alendronate): reduces bone loss, Rx: osteoporosis, Paget's disease

Foscarnet (FOSCAVIR): antiviral, Rx: cytomegalovirus

FOSCAVIR (foscarnet): antiviral, Rx: cytomegalovirus

Fosinopril (MONOPRIL): ACE inhibitor, Rx: HTN, CHF

Fosphenytoin (CEREBYX): anticonvulsant, Rx: seizures

FOSRENOL (lanthanum): phosphate binder, Rx: hyperphosphatemia in ESRD

FRAGMIN (daltaparin): LMWH, Rx: prophylaxis treatment DVT/PE, ACS

FROVA (frovatriptan): serotonin receptor agonist, Rx: migraine headaches

Furosemide (LASIX): loop diuretic, Rx: CHF, hypertension

FUZEON (enfuvirtide): antiretroviral, Rx: HIV

G

Gabapentin (NEURONTIN): anticonvulsant, Rx: seizures, postherpetic neuralgia

GABITRIL (tiagabine): anticonvulsant, Rx: partial seizures

Galantamine (RAZADYNE): cholinergic enhancer, Rx: Alzheimer's

Ganciclovir (CYTOVENE): antiviral, Rx: CMV

Gemfibrozil (LOPID): antihyperlipidemic, Rx: hypertriglyceridemia

GEMZAR (gemcitabine): antineoplastic, Rx: lung, breast, and pancreatic cancer

GENGRAF (cyclosporine): immunosuppressive, Rx: rheumatoid arthritis, psoriasis, prevention of transplant rejection

Gentamicin (GARAMYCIN): aminoglycoside antibiotic, Rx: bacterial infections

GEODON (ziprasidone): antipsychotic, Rx: schizophrenia

Glatiramir Acetate (COPAXONE): biological miscellaneous, multiple sclerosis

GLEEVEC (imatinib): antineoplastic, Rx: leukemia, gastrointestinal cancer

GLIADEL WAFER (carmustine): antineoplastic, Rx: malignant glioma, lymphomas

Glimepiride (AMARYL): oral hypoglycemic, Rx: diabetes (type 2)

Glipizide (GLUCOTROL): oral hypoglycemic, Rx: diabetes (type 2)

Glucagon: hormone, mobilizes glucose, Rx: hypoglycemia

GLUCOPHAGE (metformin): oral hypoglycemic, Rx: diabetes (type 2)

GLUCOTROL (glipizide): oral hypoglycemic, Rx: diabetes (type 2)

GLUCOVANCE (glyburide/metformin): oral hypoglycemic, Rx: diabetes (type 2)

Glyburide (DIABETA, GLYNASE): oral hypoglycemic, Rx: diabetes (type 2)

Glycopyrrolate (ROBINUL): anticholinergic, Rx: peptic ulcers

GLYNASE (glyburide): oral hypoglycemic, Rx: diabetes (type 2)

GLYSET (miglitol): oral hypoglycemic, Rx: diabetes (type 2)

GOLYTELY (polyethylene glycol-electrolyte solution): laxative, Rx: bowel cleansing

Granisetron (KYTRIL): antiemetic, Rx: chemotherapy induced nausea/vomiting

GRIFULVIN V (griseofulvin): antifungal, Rx: ringworm, onychomycosis

Griseofulvin (GRIFULVIN V): antifungal, Rx: ringworm, onychomycosis

Guaifenesin (HUMIBID, MUCINEX): expectorant, Rx: loosen bronchial secretions

Guanfacine (TENEX): antihypertensive, Rx: HTN

GYNAZOLE-1 (butoconazole): antifungal agent, vaginal, Rx: vulvovaginal candidiasis
GYNODIOL (estradiol, systemic): estrogen derivative, Rx: menopause, breast cancer

H

HALCION (triazolam): benzodiazepine hypnotic, Rx: insomnia
HALDOL (haloperidol): antiphychotic, Rx: psychotic disorders
Haloperidol (HALDOL): antipsychotic, Rx: psychotic disorders
HCT, HCTZ (hydrochlorothiazide): diuretic, Rx: HTN, water retention
HECTOROL (doxercalciferol): vitamin D supplement, Rx: hypocalcemia in renal disease, hypoparathyroidism
HEXALEN (altretamine): antineoplastic, Rx: ovarian cancer
HUMALOG (insulin lispro): hypoglycemic, Rx: diabetes
HUMIBID (guaifenesin): expectorant, Rx: loosen bronchial secretions
HUMIRA (adalimumab): immunomodulator, Rx: rheumatoid and psoriatic arthritis, ankylosing spondylitis, Crohn's disease
HUMULIN R (regular insulin): hypoglycemic, Rx: diabetes
HYCAMTIN (topotecan): antineoplastic, Rx: lung cancer
HYCODAN (hydrocodone/homatropine): narcotic antitussive
HYCOTUSS (hydrocodone/guaifenesin): narcotic antitussive/ expectorant
Hydralazine (APRESOLINE): vasodilator, Rx: HTN, CHF
Hydrochlorothiazide (HCTZ): thiazide diuretic, Rx: HTN, water retention
Hydrocodone/APAP (NORCO, LORTAB, VICODIN): narcotic analgesic compound, Rx: moderate to severe pain
HYDRODIURIL (HCTZ): diuretic, Rx: HTN, water retention
Hydromorphone (DILAUDID): opioid analgesic, Rx: moderate to severe pain
Hydroxychloroquine (PLAQUENIL): antimalarial, Rx: malaria, lupus, rheumatoid arthritis
Hydroxyurea (DROXIA, HYDREA): antineoplastic, elastogenic, Rx: melanoma, leukemia, ovarian cancer, sickle cell anemia
Hydroxyzine (ATARAX, VISTARIL): antihistamine, Rx: allergies, anxiety, sedation
Hyoscyamine (LEVSIN): antispasmodic, Rx: lower urinary tract and GI tract spasm/secretions
HYTRIN (terazosin): alpha blocker, Rx: BPH, HTN

Ibuprofen (ADVIL, MOTRIN): NSAID analgesic, Rx: arthritis, mild to moderate pain

Ibutilide (CORVERT): antiarrhythmic, Rx: atrial fibrillation, atrial flutter

Idarubicin (IDAMYCIN): antineoplastic, Rx: AML

Ifosfamide (IFEX): antineoplastic, Rx: testicular cancer

IMDUR (isosorbide mononitrate): vasodilator long acting nitrate, Rx: angina

Imipenem/Cilastatin (PRIMAXIN): carbapenem antibiotic, Rx: bacterial infections

Imipramine (TOFRANIL): tricyclic antidepressant, Rx: depression, bed wetting

IMITREX (sumatriptan): selective serotonin receptor agonist, Rx: migraine headache

IMODIUM (loperamide): slows peristalsis, Rx: diarrhea

IMURAN (azathioprine): immunosuppressant, Rx: organ transplants, lupus, rheumatoid arthritis

Indapamide (LOZOL): diuretic, Rx: HTN, edema in CHF

INDERAL, INDERAL LA (propranolol): beta blocker, Rx: HTN, angina, cardiac dysrhythmias, AMI, migraine headache

INDOCIN, INDOCIN SR (indomethacin): NSAID, Rx: arthritis

Indomethacin (INDOCIN): NSAID analgesic, Rx: arthritis

INFED (iron dextran): Rx: iron deficiency

INFERGEN (interferon alfacon-1): antiviral, Rx: hepatitis C

Infliximab (REMICADE): neutralizes tumor necrosis factor, Rx: Crohn's disease

INH (isoniazid): antibiotic, Rx: tuberculosis

INSPRA (eplerenone): aldosterone blocker, Rx: HTN, CHF

INTAL (cromolyn): anti-inflammatory, Rx: asthma

INTELENCE (etravirine): antiretroviral, Rx: HIV

INTRON A (interferon alpha-2b): interferon, Rx: chronic hepatitis B/C, leukemia, lymphoma

INVEGA (paliperidone): antipsychotic, Rx: schizophrenia

INVIRASE (saquinavir): protease inhibitor antiretroviral, Rx: HIV

Irinotecan (CAMPTOSAR): antineoplastic, Rx: colon and rectal cancer

IONAMIN (phentermine): anorexiant stimulant, Rx: obesity

Ipecac: detoxification agent, Rx: overdose/poisoning

Ipratropium (ATROVENT): bronchodilator, Rx: COPD
ISENTRESS (raltegravir): antiretroviral, Rx: HIV
ISMO (isosorbide mononitrate): vasodilator, Rx: angina
Isoniazid: antibiotic, Rx: tuberculosis
Isoproterenol: beta bronchodilator, Rx: asthma, COPD
ISOPTIN SR (verapamil): calcium channel blocker, Rx: angina, HTN, PSVT prophylaxis, headache
ISOPTO CARPINE OPTH (pilocarpine): cholinergic miotic, Rx: glaucoma
Isosorbide dinitrate (ISORDIL): nitrate vasodilator, Rx: angina
Isosorbide mononitrate (IMDUR, ISMO, MONOKET): long-acting nitrate, Rx: angina
Isradipine (DYNACIRC): calcium channel blocker, Rx: HTN
Itraconazole (SPORANOX): antifungal, Rx: fungal infections

J

JANUMET (sitagliptin/metformin): oral hypoglycemics, Rx: diabetes (type 2)
JANUVIA (sitagliptin): oral hypoglycemic, Rx: diabetes (type 2)
JOLIVETTE (norethindrone): contraceptive, progestin, Rx: amenorrhea, prevent pregnancy, endometriosis
JUNEL (ethinyl estradiol and norethindrone): contraceptive, Rx: prevent pregnancy, acne, menopause

K

KADIAN (morphine ER): opioid analgesic, Rx: severe pain
KALETRA (lopinavir/ritonavir): antiretrovirals, Rx: HIV
KAOPECTATE (bismuth): gastrointestinal, Rx: indigestion, diarrhea
Kanamycin (KANTREX): aminoglycoside antibiotic, Rx: bacterial infection
KAPIDEX (dexlansoprazole): proton pump inhibitor, Rx: GERD, erosive esophagitis
KAYEXALATE (sodium polystyrene sulfonate): antidote, Rx: hyperkalemia
K-DUR (potassium): electrolyte, Rx: hypokalemia
KEFLEX (cephalexin): cephalosporin antibiotic, Rx: bacterial infections
KEPPRA (levatiracetam): anticonvulsant, Rx: seizures

KERLONE (betaxolol): beta-1 blocker, Rx: HTN
KETEK (telithromycin): ketolide antibiotic, Rx: community acquired PNA
Ketoconazole (NIZORAL): antifungal agent, Rx: fungal infections
Ketoprofen: NSAID analgesic, Rx: arthritis
Ketorolac (TORADOL): NSAID analgesic, Rx: acute pain
Ketotifen OPTH (ZADITOR): antihistamine, anti-inflammatory, Rx: allergic conjunctivitis
KINERET (anakinra): antirheumatic, disease modifying, Rx: rheumatoid arthritis
KLONOPIN (clonazepam): benzodiazepine hypnotic, Rx: seizures, panic disorder
KLOR-CON (potassium): electrolyte, Rx: hypokalemia
KOGENATE (antihemophilic Factor VIII): Rx: hemophilia
KONSYL (psyllium): bulk-forming laxative, Rx: constipation
KRISTALOSE (lactulose): ammonium detoxicant, laxative, Rx: constipation
KUTRASE (pancreatin): pancreatic enzymes replacement in CF, chronic pancreatitis
KWELL (lindane): parasiticide, Rx: lice, scabies
KYTRIL (granisetron): antiemetic, Rx: chemotherapy induced nausea/vomiting

L

Labetalol (TRANDATE): beta blocker, Rx: HTN
LAC-HYDRIN (ammonium lactate): emollient, Rx: dry, itchy skin
LACRI-LUBE OPTH (white petrolatum/mineral oil): Rx: ophthalmic lubrication
LACRISERT (hydroxypropyl): opthalmic lubricant, Rx: dry eyes
Lactulose (CEPHULAC): hyperosmotic laxative, Rx: constipation, encephalopathy
LAMICTAL (lamotrigine): anticonvulsant, Rx: seizures, bipolar disorder
LAMISIL (terbinafine): antifungal, Rx: fungal infections
Lamivudine (EPIVIR): antiviral, Rx: HIV
Lamotrigine (LAMICTAL): anticonvulsant, Rx: seizures, bipolar disorder
LANOXIN (digoxin): cardiac glycoside, Rx: CHF, atrial fibrillation

Lansoprazole (PREVACID): gastric acid pump inhibitor, Rx: ulcers, GERD

Lantus (insulin glargine): hypoglycemic, Rx: diabetes

Lariam (mefloquine): antimalarial agent

Lasix (furosemide): loop diuretic, Rx: HTN, CHF

Leflunomide (ARAVA): immunomodulator, anti-inflammatory, Rx: rheumatoid arthritis

Lescol (fluvastatin): statin, Rx: hypercholesterolemia

Lessina (ethinyl estradiol and levonorgestrel): contraceptive, Rx: prevent pregnancy

Leukeran (chlorambucil): antineoplastic, Rx: leukemia, lymphoma, Hodgkin's disease

Leucovorin: vitamin, Rx: methotrexate toxicity, megaloblastic anemia

Leuprolide (LUPRON): hormone, Rx: endometriosis, advanced prostate cancer

Levalbuterol (XOPENEX): inhaled beta2, bronchodilator, Rx: COPD, asthma

Levamisole (ERGAMISOLE): immunostimulant, Rx: colon cancer

Levaquin (levofloxacin): antibiotic, Rx: pneumonia, COPD, UTI

Levetiracetam (KEPPRA): anticonvulsant, Rx: seizures

Levatol (penbutolol): beta blocker, Rx: hypertension

Levbid (hyoscyamine): anticholinergic agent, Rx: peptic ulcer, colic, GI disorders

Levemir (insulin detemir): hypoglycemic, Rx: diabetes

Levitra (vardenafil): vasodilator, Rx: erectile dysfunction

Levlen (ethinyl estradiol and levonorgestrel): contraceptive, Rx: prevent pregnancy

Levlin (ethinyl estradiol/levonorgestrel): oral contraceptive

Levobunolol OPTH (BETAGAN): beta blocker, Rx: glaucoma

Levodopa/carbidopa (SINEMET): dopamine precursor, Rx: Parkinson's disease

Levofloxacin (LEVAQUIN): fluoroquinolone antibiotic, Rx: bacterial infections

Levora (levonorgestrel/estradiol): oral contraceptive

Levothroid (levothyroxine): thyroid hormone, Rx: hypothyroidism

Levothyroxine (LEVOTHROID, LEVOXYL, SYNTHROID): thyroid hormone, Rx: hypothyroidism

Levoxyl (levothyroxine): thyroid hormone, Rx: hypothyroidism

Levsin, Levsinex (hyoscyamine): antispasmodic, Rx: lower urinary tract and GI tract spasm/secretions

LEXAPRO (escitalopram): SSRI antidepressant, Rx: depression, anxiety disorder

LEXIVA (fosamprenavir): antiretroviral, Rx: HIV

LIBRIUM (chlordiazepoxide): benzodiazepine, Rx: anxiety, alcohol withdrawal

Lindane (KWELL): parasiticide, Rx: scabies, lice

Liothyronine (CYTOMEL): thyroid hormone, Rx: hypothyroidism

Liotrix (THYROLAR): thyroid hormone, Rx: hypothyroidism

LIPITOR (atorvastatin): statin, Rx: hypercholesterolemia, CHD

LIPRAM UL (pancrelipase): pancreatic enzymes replacement, Rx: chronic pancreatitis, cystic fibrosis

Lisinopril (PRINIVIL, ZESTRIL): ACE inhibitor, Rx: HTN, CHF, AMI

Lisinopril/HCTZ (ZESTORETIC): ACE inhibitor, Rx: HTN, CHF, AMI

Lithium (LITHOBID): antipsychotic, Rx: bipolar disorder

LITHOBID (lithium): antipsychotic, Rx: bipolar disorder

LODRANE 12D (brompheniramine/pseudoephedrine): antihistamine/decongestant, Rx: allergies, common cold

LOESTRIN (ethinyl estradiol/norethindrone): oral contraceptive

LOMOTIL (diphenoxylate/atropine): opioid congener, Rx: diarrhea

LONOX (diphenoxylate/atropine): opioid congener, Rx: diarrhea

LO/OVRAL (ethinyl estradiol/norgestrel): oral contraceptive

Loperamide (IMODIUM): slows peristalsis, Rx: diarrhea

LOPID (gemfibrozil): antihyperlipidemic, Rx: hypertriglyceridemia

Lopinavir (KALETRA): antiviral, Rx: HIV, AIDS

LOPRESSOR (metoprolol): beta-1 blocker, Rx: hypertension

LOPROX (ciclopirox): antifungal, Rx: ringworm, candida

Loratadine (CLARITIN): antihistamine, Rx: allergies

Lorazepam (ATIVAN): benzodiazepine hypnotic, Rx: anxiety, status epilepticus

LORCET 10/650, **LORCET HD, LORCET PLUS** (hydrocodone/ APAP): opioid analgesic compound, Rx: mild to moderate pain

LORTAB (hydrocodone/APAP): narcotic analgesic

Losartan (COZAAR): angiotensin receptor blocker, Rx: HTN, diabetic nephropathy

LOTENSIN (benazepril): ACE inhibitor, Rx: HTN, CHF

LOTENSIN HCT (benazepril/HCTZ): ACE inhibitor/diuretic, Rx: HTN

LOTREL (amlodipine/benazepril): calcium channel blocker/ACE inhibitor, Rx: HTN

LOTRONEX (alosetron): antidiarrheal, Rx: irritable bowel syndrome

Lovastatin (MEVACOR): statin, Rx: hypercholesterolemia, CHD

LOVENOX (enoxaparin): LMWH, Rx: prophylaxis/tx DVT/PE, ACS
LOW-OGESTREL (ethinyl estradiol and norgestrel): contraceptive, Rx: prevent pregnancy, "morning after pill"
Loxapine (LOXITANE): antipsychotic, Rx: schizophrenia
LOXITANE (loxapine): antipsychotic, Rx: schizophrenia
LOZOL (indapamide): diuretic, Rx: HTN, edema in CHF
LUCENTIS (ranibizumab): blood vessel growth inhibitor, Rx: macular degeneration
LUMIGAN OPTH (bimatoprost): lowers intraocular pressure, Rx: glaucoma
LUNESTA (eszopiclone): sedative, Rx: insomnia
LUPRON DEPOT (leuprolide): hormone, Rx: endometriosis, prostrate cancer
LUVOX (fluvoxamine): SSRI antidepressant, Rx: obsessive-compulsive disorder, anxiety
LYRICA (pregabalin): anticonvulsant, Rx: partial seizures, neuropathic pain

M

MACROBID (nitrofurantoin): nitrofuran antibiotic, Rx: UTI
MACRODANTIN (nitrofurantoin): nitrofuran antibiotic, Rx: UTI
MALARONE (atovaquone/proguanil): antimalarial agents, Rx: malaria prevention/treatment
Malathion (OVIDE): organophosphate insecticide, Rx: head lice
Mannitol (OSMITROL): osmotic diuretic, Rx: cerebral edema, IOP
Maprotiline (LUDIOMIL): tetracyclic antidepressant, Rx: depression, bipolar disorder, anxiety
MARINOL (dronabinol): appetite stimulant, Rx: weight loss in cancer, AIDS
MAVIK (trandolapril): ACE inhibitor, Rx: HTN, CHF post MI
MAXAIR (pirbuterol): inhaled beta$_2$ stimulant, Rx: asthma, COPD
MAXALT (rizatriptan): selective serotonin receptor agonist, Rx: migraine headaches
MAXIDEX OPTH (dexamethasone): corticosteroid, Rx: corneal injury, allergic conjunctivitis
MAXITROL OPTH (neomycin/polymyxin/dexamethasone): antibiotics/steroid, Rx: eye infection/inflammation
MAXZIDE (triamterene/HCTZ): diuretics, Rx: HTN, water retention

MEBARAL (mephobarbital): barbiturate sedative, Rx: epilepsy, anxiety

Mebendazole (VERMOX): anthelmintic, Rx: intestinal worms

Meclizine (ANTIVERT): antinauseant, Rx: motion sickness

Meclofenamate: NSAID analgesic, Rx: arthritis, acute pain

MEDROL (methylprednisolone): glucocorticoid, Rx: adrenal insufficiency, allergies, RA

Medroxyprogesterone (PROVERA): progestin hormone, Rx: endometriosis, amenorrhea, uterine bleeding, contraception

MEFOXIN (cefoxitin): cephalosporin antibiotic, Rx: bacterial infections

Mefloquine (LARIAM): antimalarial, Rx: prevention and treatment of malaria

Megestrol (MEGACE): progestin, appetite stimulant, Rx: anorexia with AIDS, antineoplastic, Rx: breast cancer, endometrial cancer

Meloxicam (MOBIC): NSAID analgesic, Rx: arthritis

Meperidine (DEMEROL): opioid analgesic, Rx: moderate to severe pain

MEPHYTON (vitamin K-1): Rx: coagulation disorders

Meprobamate (MILTOWN): antianxiety agent, Rx: anxiety disorders

MEPRON (atovaquone): antiprotozoal, Rx: prophylaxis and treatment for pneumocystic carinii pneumonia in AIDS

Mercaptopurine (PURINETHOL): antineoplastic, Rx: leukemia

MERIDIA (sibutramine): stimulant, Rx: obesity

MERREM (meropenem): carbapenem antibiotic, Rx: bacterial infections

Mesalamine (ASACOL, PENTASA): anti-inflammatory agent, Rx: ulcerative colitis

MESTINON (pyridostigmine): anticholinesterase, Rx: myasthenia gravis

METADATE CD, ER (methylphenidate): stimulant, Rx: ADHD, narcolepsy

METAGLIP (glipizide/metformin): oral hypoglycemics, Rx: diabetes (type 2)

Metaproterenol (ALUPENT): beta$_2$ agonist bronchodilator, Rx: COPD, asthma

Metformin (GLUCOPHAGE): oral hypoglycemic, Rx: diabetes (type 2)

Methadone (DOLOPHINE): opioid analgesic, Rx: moderate to severe pain, opiate withdrawal

METHADOSE (methadone): analgesic, opioid, Rx: detoxification of opioid addiction

Methenamine (URISED, UREX): antibiotic, Rx: UTI prophylaxis
METHERGINE (methylergonovine): increases uterine contractions, Rx: uterine contraction/bleeding
Methimazole (TAPAZOLE): Rx: antithyroid; Rx: hyperthyroidism
Methocarbamol (ROBAXIN): skeletal muscle relaxant
Methotrexate: antineoplastic, Rx: psoriasis, cancer, rheumatoid arthritis
Methsuximide (CELONTIN): anticonvulsant, Rx: absence seizure
Methyldopa (ALDOMET): centrally acting antihypertensive, Rx: HTN
Methylphenidate (RITALIN): stimulant, Rx: ADHD, narcolepsy
Methylprednisolone (MEDROL): glucocorticoid, Rx: adrenal insufficiency, allergies, RA
Metoclopramide (REGLAN): improves gastric emptying, Rx: heartburn, diabetic gastroparesis
Metolazone (ZAROXOLYN): thiazide diuretic, Rx: HTN, fluid retention
Metoprolol (LOPRESSOR, TOPROL-XL): beta-1 blocker, Rx: HTN, angina, dysrhythmias
Metronidazole (FLAGYL): antibiotic, Rx: bacterial infections
MEVACOR (lovastatin): statin, Rx: hypercholesterolemia, CHD
Mexiletine (MEXITIL): antiarrhythmic, Rx: ventricular dysrhythmias
MEXITIL (mexiletine): antiarrhythmic, Rx: ventricular dysrhythmias
MIACALCIN (calcitonin-salmon): bone resorption inhibitor hormone, Rx: hypercalcemia, Paget's disease, osteoporosis
MICARDIS (telmisartan): angiotensin II receptor antagonist, Rx: HTN
Miconazole (MONISTAT): antifungal, Rx: candidiasis
MICRO-K (potassium): electrolyte, Rx: hypokalemia
MICROZIDE (HCTZ): thiazide diuretic, Rx: HTN, water retention
MIDAMOR (amiloride): potassium-sparing diuretic, Rx: HTN, CHF
Midazolam: benzodiazepine hypnotic, Rx: anxiety before surgery
Midodrine (PROAMATINE): vasopressor, Rx: orthostatic hypotension
MIDRIN (isometheptene, dichloralphenazone, APAP): vasoconstrictor/sedative/analgesic, Rx: migraines
MINIPRESS (prazosin): alpha-1 blocker, Rx: hypertension
MINITRAN (transdermal nitroglycerin): nitrate, Rx: angina
MINOCIN (minocycline): tetracycline antibiotic, Rx: bacterial infections, acne
Minocycline (MINOCIN): tetracycline antibiotic, Rx: bacterial infections, acne
Minoxidil: vasodilator, Rx: severe HTN

MIRALAX (polyethylene glycol): osmotic laxative, Rx: constipation

MIRAPEX (pramipexole): dopamine agonist, Rx: Parkinson's disease, restless legs syndrome

MIRCERA (methoxypolyethyleneglycol-epoetin): increases RBC production, Rx: anemia in chronic renal failure

Mirtazapine (REMERON): antidepressant, Rx: depression

Misoprostol (CYTOTEC): antiulcer, Rx: NSAID-induced gastric ulcers

MOBIC (meloxicam): NSAID analgesic, Rx: arthritis

Modafinil (PROVIGIL): wakefulness-promoting agent, Rx: narcolepsy, daytime sleepiness

MODURETIC (amiloride/HCTZ): diuretics, Rx: HTN, fluid retention

Moexipril (UNIVASC): ACE inhibitor, Rx: HTN

MONOCAL (fluoride, calcium): mineral supplement

MONOKET (isosorbide mononitrate): long acting nitrate, Rx: angina

MONOPRIL (fosinopril): ACE inhibitor, Rx: HTN, CHF

MONUROL (fosfomycin): antibiotic, Rx: UTI

Morphine sulfate (MS CONTIN): opioid analgesic, Rx: moderate to severe pain

MOTOFEN (difenoxin/atropine): decreases intestinal motility, Rx: diarrhea

Moxifloxacin (AVELOX): fluoroquinolone antibiotic, Rx: bacterial infections

MS CONTIN (morphine ER): narcotic analgesic, Rx: moderate to severe pain

MUCINEX (guaifenesin): expectorant, Rx: loosen bronchial secretions

MYCELEX 3 (butoconazole): vaginal antifungal, Rx: yeast infection

MYCOBUTIN (rifabutin): antibiotic, Rx: mycobacterium avium complex in HIV

Mycophenolate (CELLCEPT): immunosuppressant, Rx: organ transplants

MYCOSTATIN (nystatin): antifungal, Rx: candidiasis

MYLERAN (busulfan): alkylating agent, Rx: leukemia

MYSOLINE (primidone): anticonvulsant, Rx: seizures

N

Nabumetone (RELAFEN): NSAID analgesic, Rx: arthritis

Nadolol (CORGARD): beta blocker, Rx: HTN, angina

Nafcillin: penicillin antibiotic, Rx: bacterial infection

Naftifine (NAFTIN): antifungal, Rx: fungal infections

Nalbuphine (NUBAIN): opioid agonist-antagonist analgesic, Rx: pain relief, pruritis

Naltrexone (REVIA): narcotic antagonist, Rx: narcotic or alcohol addiction

NAMENDA (memantine): NMDA antagonist, Rx: Alzheimer's disease

Naphazoline OPTH (NAPHCON): vasoconstrictor, Rx: relief of eye redness, irritation

NAPHCON OPTH (naphazoline): vasoconstrictor, Rx: relief of eye redness, irritation

NAPROSYN (naproxen): NSAID analgesic, Rx: arthritis, pain, inflammation, headache

NARDIL (phenelzine): MAO inhibitor, Rx: depression, bulimia

NASACORT AQ (triamcinolone): nasal corticosteroid, Rx: allergic rhinitis

NASALCROM (cromolyn): nasal anti-inflammatory agent, Rx: allergic rhinitis

NASAREL (flunisolide): nasal corticosteroid, Rx: allergic rhinitis

NASONEX (mometasone): nasal corticosteroid, Rx: allergic rhinitis

NATRECOR (nesiritide): b-type natriuretic peptide vasodilator, Rx: CHF

NAVANE (thiothixene): antipsychotic, Rx: schizophrenia

NECON (ethinyl estradiol and norethindrone): contraceptive, Rx: prevent pregnancy, acne, menopause

Nefazodone (SERZONE): antidepressant, Rx: depression

Nelfinavir (VIRACEPT): protease inhibitor antiretroviral, Rx: HIV

NEMBUTAL (pentobarbital): barbiturate, Rx: insomnia, sleep induction, status epilepticus

Neomycin: aminoglycoside antibiotic, Rx: preoperative bowel preparation, encephalopathy

NEOPROFEN (ibuprofen lysine): Rx: closure patent ductus arteriosus in premature infants

NEORAL (cyclosporine): immunosuppressant, Rx: organ transplant

NEPHROCAPS (vitamins): vitamin supplement, Rx: uremia, renal failure

NEULASTA (pegfilgrastim): colony stimulating factor, Rx: myelosuppressive chemotherapy

NEURONTIN (gabapentin): anticonvulsant, Rx: seizures, postherpetic neuralgia

NEUPOGEN (filgrastim): white blood cell stimulator,

Nevirapine (VIRAMUNE): antiretroviral, Rx: HIV

NEXIUM (esomeprazole): protein pump inhibitor, Rx: esophagitis, GERD, ulcers

Niacin (vitamin B-3): nicotinic acid, Rx: hypercholesterolemia, hypertriglyceridemia

NIACOR (niacin): vitamin B-3, Rx: hypercholesterolemia, hypertriglyceridemia

NIASPAN (niacin slow release): vitamin B-3, Rx: hypercholesterolemia, hypertriglyceridemia

Nicardipine (CARDENE): calcium channel blocker, Rx: angina, HTN

NICODERM (transdermal nicotine): Rx: smoking cessation

NICOMIDE-T (niacinamide): vitamin, water soluable, Rx: pellagra, acne

NICORETTE (nicotine): smoking cessation aid, Rx: relief of nicotine withdrawal

Nicotinic Acid (niacin): vitamin B-3, Rx: hypercholesterolemia, hypertriglyceridemia

NICOTROL Inhaler (nicotine): Rx: smoking cessation

NICOTROL NS (nicotine): Rx: smoking cessation

Nifedipine (PROCARDIA, ADALAT): calcium channel blocker, Rx: angina, HTN

NIFEREX, NIFEREX-150 (iron): mineral, Rx: anemia

NILANDRON (nilutamide): antiandrogen, Rx: prostate cancer

Nimodipine (NIMOTOP): calcium channel blocker, Rx: improves neurological deficits after subarachnoid hemorrhage

NIMOTOP (nimodipine): calcium channel blocker, Rx: improves neurological deficits after subarachnoid hemorrhage

Nisoldipine (SULAR): calcium channel blocker, Rx: HTN

NITRO-DUR (nitroglycerin): transdermal nitrate, Rx: angina

Nitrofurantoin (macrodantin): antibacterial agent, Rx: UTI

Nitroglycerin (NITROSTAT): vasodilator, Rx: angina

NITROLINGUAL SPRAY (nitroglycerin): nitrate, Rx: angina

NITROMIST (nitroglycerin): vasodilator lingual spray, Rx: angina

NITROSTAT (nitroglycerin): vasodilator, Rx: angina

NIX (permethrin): parasiticide, Rx: head lice

Nizatidine (AXID): histamine-2 antagonist, Rx: ulcers, GERD

NIZORAL (ketoconazole): antifungal agent, Rx: fungal infections

NORCO (hydrocodone/APAP): narcotic analgesic compound, Rx: moderate to severe pain

NORDETTE (ethinyl estradiol and levonorgestrel): contraceptive, Rx: prevent pregnancy

NORFLEX (orphenadrine): skeletal muscle relaxant
Norfloxacin (NOROXIN): fluoroquinolone antibiotic, Rx: bacterial infections
NORGESIC (orphenadrine): skeletal muscle relaxant
NORINYL (ethinyl estradiol and norethindrone): contraceptive, Rx: prevent pregnancy, acne, menopause
NOROXIN (norfloxacin): fluoroquinolone antibiotic, Rx: bacterial infections
NORPACE, NORPACE CR (disopyramide): antiarrhythmic, Rx: ventricular dysrhythmias
NORPRAMIN (desipramine): a tricyclic antidepressant, Rx: depression
NOR-QD (norethindrone): contraceptive, Rx: amenorrhea, endometriosis, prevent pregnancy
NORTREL (ethinyl estradiol and norethindrone): contraceptive, Rx: prevent pregnancy, acne, menopause
Nortriptyline (PAMELOR): a tricyclic antidepressant
NORVASC (amlodipine): calcium blocker, Rx: HTN, angina
NORVIR (ritonavir): protease inhibitor antiretroviral, Rx: HIV
NOVANTRONE (mitoxantrone): antineoplastic, Rx: prostate cancer, leukemia, multiple sclerosis
NOVOLIN R (regular insulin): hypoglycemic, Rx: diabetes
NOVOLOG (insulin aspart): hypoglycemic, Rx: diabetes
NOVOLOG MIX 70/30 (insulin mixture): hypoglycemic, Rx: diabetes
NUBAIN (nalbuphine): opioid agonist-antagonist analgesic, Rx: pain relief, pruritis
NUVIGIL (armodafinil): CNS stimulant, Rx: narcolepsy, shift-work sleep disorder
Nystatin (MYCOSTATIN): antifungal, Rx: candidiasis
NYSTOP (nystatin): antifungal, Rx: candidiasis

O

Octreotide (SANDOSTATIN): antidiarrheal, growth inhibitor, Rx: acromegaly, diarrhea associated with carcinoid and intestinal tumors
OCUFLOX OPTH (ofloxacin): fluoroquinolone antibiotic, Rx: conjunctivitis, corneal ulcers
Ofloxacin (FLOXIN): fluoroquinolone antibiotic, Rx: bacterial infections

Olanzapine (ZYPREXA): antipsychotic, Rx: schizophrenia, bipolar disorder

Olopatadine (PATANOL): antihistamine, Rx: allergic conjunctivitis

Olsalazine (DIPENTUM): salicylate, Rx: ulcerative colitis

Omeprazole (PRILOSEC): suppresses gastric acid secretion, Rx: ulcers, esophagitis, GERD

OMNARIS (ciclesonide): intranasal steroid, Rx: allergic rhinitis

OMNICEF (cefdinir): cephalosporin antibiotic, Rx: bacterial infections

OMNIHIST LA (chlorpheniramine/phenylephrine/methscopalamine): antihistamine/decongestant, Rx: rhinitis, colds

Ondansetron (ZOFRAN): antinauseant, Rx: nausea and vomiting secondary to chemotherapy, radiation, and surgery

OPANA (oxymorphone): opioid analgesic, Rx: moderate to severe pain

Opium Tincture (morphine): opioid analgesic, Rx: diarrhea

OPTIVAR OPTH (azelastine): antihistamine, Rx: allergic conjunctivitis

ORAMORPH SR (morphine sulfate SR): opioid analgesic, Rx: moderate to severe pain

ORENCIA (abatacept): immunomodulator, Rx: rheumatoid arthritis

ORINASE (tolbutamide): oral hypoglycemic, Rx: diabetes (type 2)

Orphenadrine (NORFLEX): skeletal muscle relaxant

ORTHO EVRA (ethinyl estradiol and norelgestromin): contraceptive, Rx: prevent pregnancy

ORTHO TRI-CYCLEN (ethinyl estradiol and norgestimate): contraceptive, Rx: prevent pregnancy, acne

ORTHO-CEPT (ethinyl estradiol and desogestrel): contraceptive, Rx: prevent pregnancy

ORTHO-CYCLEN (ethinyl estradiol and norgestimate): contraceptive, Rx: prevent pregnancy, acne

ORTHO-EST (piperazine estrone sulfate): estrogen derivative, Rx: menopause, osteoporosis

ORTHO-NOVUM (ethinyl estradiol and norethindrone): contraceptive, Rx: prevent pregnancy, acne, menopause

OS-CAL (calcium, vitamin D): calcium salt, electrolyte supplement, Rx: antacid, dietary supplement

OVCON (ethinyl estradiol and norethindrone): contraceptive, Rx: prevent pregnancy, acne, menopause

OVIDE (malathon): antiparasitic/scabicidal agent, Rx: head lice and their ova

Oxacillin: penicillin class antibiotic, Rx: bacterial infections

Oxandrolone (OXANDRIN): anabolic steroid, Rx: osteoporosis, promotes weight gain
Oxaprozin (DAYPRO): NSAID analgesic, Rx: arthritis
Oxazepam (SERAX): benzodiazepine hypnotic, Rx: anxiety, alcohol withdrawal
Oxcarbazepine (TRILEPTAL): anticonvulsant, Rx: partial seizures
Oxybutynin (DITROPAN): anticholinergic, antispasmodic, Rx: overactive bladder
Oxycodone (ROXICODNE, OXYCONTIN): opioid analgesic, Rx: moderate to severe pain
Oxycodone/ASA (PERCODAN): opioid analgesic/aspirin, Rx: moderate to severe pain
Oxycodone w/APAP (ENDOCET, PERCOCET, TYLOX): opioid analgesic/APAP, Rx: moderate to severe pain
OXYCONTIN (oxycodone SR): opioid analgesic, Rx: moderate to severe pain
OXYFAST (oxycodone): opioid analgesic, Rx: moderate to severe pain
Oxymetazoline (AFRIN): nasal decongestant, Rx: sinusitis, cold
Oxymetholone (ANADROL-50): anabolic steroid/androgen, Rx: anemia
Oxytocin (PITOCIN): stimulates uterine contractions, Rx: induction of labor
OXYTROL (oxybutynin): transdermal anticholinergic, antispasmodic, Rx: overactive bladder

P

PACERONE (amiodarone): antiarrhythmic, Rx: dysrhythmias
Paclitaxel (TAXOL): antineoplastic, Rx: ovarian cancer, breast cancer, Kaposi's sarcoma
Palivizumab (SYNAGIS): antiviral antibody, Rx: respiratory syncytial virus prevention
PAMELOR (nortriptyline): tricyclic antidepressant, Rx: depression
PANCREASE, PANCREASE MT (pancrelipase): pancreatic enzymes replacement, Rx: chronic pancreatitis, cystic fibrosis
Pancrelipase (CREON 5, PANCREASE): pancreatic enzymes replacement, Rx: chronic pancreatitis, cystic fibrosis
PANGESTYME (pancrelipase): pancreatic enzymes replacement, Rx: chronic pancreatitis, cystic fibrosis

Pantoprazole (PROTONIX): suppresses gastic acid, Rx: ulcers, GERD
PARAPLATIN (carboplatin): antineoplastic, Rx: ovarian cancer
PARCOPA (carbidopa/levodopa): dopamine precursors, Rx: Parkinson's disease
PAREGORIC (morphine): opioid analgesic, Rx: diarrhea
Paricalcitol (ZEMPLAR): vitamin D, Rx: hyperparathyroidism in chronic kidney disease
PARNATE (tranylcypromine): MAO inhibitor, Rx: depression
Paroxetine (PAXIL): SSRI antidepressant, Rx: depression, OCD, anxiety, PTSD
PASER (aminosalicylic acid): antibacterial, Rx: tuberculosis
PATANASE (olopatadine): nasal antihistamine, Rx: allergic rhinitis
PATANOL OPTH (olopatadine): antihistamine, Rx: allergic conjunctivitis
PAXIL (paroxetine): SSRI antidepressant, Rx: depression, OCD, anxiety, PTSD
PEDIAFLOR (fluoride): mineral, Rx: osteoporosis, dental caries
PEDIAPRED (prednisolone): glucocorticoid, Rx: allergies, arthritis, multiple sclerosis
PEGANONE (ethotoin): anticonvulsant, Rx: seizures
PEGASYS (peginterferon alfa-2a): interferon, Rx: chronic hepatitis B and C
PEGINTRON (interferon alfa-2b): antiviral, Rx: chronic hepatitis C
Pemirolast OPTH (ALAMAST): anti-inflammatory, Rx: allergic conjunctivitis
Pemoline (CYLERT): stimulant, Rx: ADHD
Penbutolol (LEVATOL): beta blocker, Rx: HTN
Penicillamine (CUPRIMINE, DEPEN): chelator, antirheumatic, Rx: heavy metal poisoning, Wilson's disease, arthritis, cystinuria
Penicillin (VEETIDS): penicillin antibiotic, Rx: bacterial infection
Pentamidine (PENTAM 300): antiprotozoal, Rx: P. carinii pneumonia
PENTASA (mesalamine): anti-inflammatory, Rx: ulcerative colitis
Pentazocine (TALWIN): opioid agonist-antagonist analgesic, Rx: moderate to severe pain
Pentazocine/Naloxone (TALWIN NX): opioid analgesic compound, Rx: pain

Pentazocine/APAP (TALACEN): opioid analgesic/APAP compound

Pentobarbital (NEMBUTAL): barbiturate hypnotic, Rx: insomnia, status epilepticus

Pentostatin (NIPENT): antineoplastic, Rx: hairy cell leukemia

Pentoxifylline (TRENTAL): reduces blood viscosity, Rx: intermittent claudication

PEPCID, PEPCID AC (famotidine): histamine-2 blocker, reduces gastric acid, Rx: ulcers, GERD

PERCOCET (oxycodone/APAP): opioid analgesic, Rx: moderate to severe pain

PERCODAN (oxycodone/aspirin): opioid analgesic, Rx: moderate to severe pain

PERFOROMIST (formoterol): beta$_2$ adenergic agonist, long acting, Rx: asthma, COPD

PERIACTIN (cyproheptadine): antihistamine, Rx: allergies

PERI-COLACE (docusate/senna): stool softener/laxative, Rx: constipation

Perindopril (ACEON): ACE inhibitor, Rx: HTN, CAD

Permethrin (ELIMITE, ACTICIN, NIX): parasiticide, Rx: head lice, scabies

Perphenazine (TRILAFON): anitpsychotic, Rx: schizophrenia, hiccoughs

PERSANTINE (dipyridamole): platelet inhibitor, Rx: blood clots after heart valve replacement

Phenazopyridine (PYRIDIUM): urinary tract analgesic, Rx: relief of pain on urination

Phenelzine (NARDIL): MAO inhibitor, Rx: depression

PHENERGAN (promethazine): sedative/antiemetic, Rx: rhinitis, urticaria, nausea and vomiting

Phenobarbital: barbiturate sedative, Rx: sedative, anticonvulsant

Phentermine (ADIPEX-P): amphetamine, Rx: obesity

Phenyl Salicylate/methenamine (PROSED/DS, UROGESIC BLUE): analgesic, Rx: urinary tract discomfort, cystitis, urethritis

Phenylephrine (NEO-SYNEPHRINE, SUDAFED PE): decongestant, Rx: colds, allergies

Phenytoin (DILANTIN): anticonvulsant, Rx: epilepsy

PHISOHEX (hexachlorophene): bacteriostatic skin cleanser

PhosLo (calcium): antidote, calcium salt, phosphate binder, Rx: hyperphosphatemia

PHRENILIN, PHRENILIN FORTE (butalbital/acetaminophen):

Phytonadione (AQUAMEPHYTON): vitamin K1, Rx: coagulation disorders

Pilocarpine (SALAGEN): cholinergic, Rx: dry mouth, Sjogren's syndrome

Pilocarpine OPTH (ISOPTO CARPINE, PILOCAR): cholinergic miotic, Rx: glaucoma

PIMA (potassium iodide): expectorant, Rx: asthma, bronchitis

Pindolol (VISKEN): beta blocker, Rx: HTN

Pioglitazone (ACTOS): oral hypoglycemic, Rx: diabetes (type 2)

Piperacillin (PIPRACIL): penicillin antibiotic, Rx: bacterial infections

Pirbuterol (MAXAIR): beta bronchodilator, Rx: asthma, COPD

Piroxicam (FELDENE): NSAID analgesic, Rx: arthritis

PLAQUENIL (hydroxychloroquine): antimalarial agent, Rx: malaria, rheumatoid arthritis, lupus

PLAVIX (clopidogrel): platelet inhibitor, Rx: MI, stroke, atherosclerosis

PLETAL (cilostazol): platelet inhibitor, Rx: intermittent claudication

PNEUMOTUSSIN (guaifenesin/hydrocodone): expectorant/opioid antitussive, Rx: cough

PODOCON-25 (podophyllin): cytotoxic, Rx: genital warts

Podofilox (CONDYLOX): destroys warts, Rx: anogenital warts

Podophyllin (PODOCON-25): cytotoxic agent, Rx: genital warts

Polyethylene glycol (MIRALAX): osmotic laxative, Rx: constipation

Polymyxin B (Poly-Rx) polymixin B sulfate, antibiotic, Rx: acute infections

POLYTRIM OPTH (trimethoprim/polymyxin): antibiotic compound, Rx: eye infections

PONSTEL (mefenamic acid): NSAID analgesic, Rx: mild to moderate pain

Posaconazole (NOXAFIL): antifungal, Rx: fungal infections

Potassium citrate (UROCIT-K): urinary alkalinizer, Rx: kidney stones

Potassium iodide (PIMA): expectorant, Rx: asthma, bronchitis

Pramipexole (MIRAPEX): dopamine agonist, Rx: Parkinson's disease, restless leg syndrome

PRANDIMET (repaglinide/metformin): oral hypoglycemics, Rx: diabetes (type 2)

PRANDIN (repaglinide): oral hypoglycemia, Rx: diabetes (type 2)

PRAVACHOL (pravastatin): statin, Rx: hypercholesterolemia, CAD

Pravastatin (PRAVACHOL): statin, Rx: hypercholesterolemia, CAD

Prazosin (MINIPRESS): alpha-1 blocker, vasodilator, Rx: HTN

PRECOSE (acarbose): delays carbohydrate digestion, Rx: diabetes mellitus (type 2)

Prednisolone (ORAPRED, PRELONE): glucocorticoid, Rx: adrenal insufficiency, allergies, RA, lupus, COPD

Prednisone (DELTASONE): glucocorticoid, Rx: adrenal insufficiency, allergies, RA, lupus, COPD

PRELONE (prednisolone): glucocorticoid, Rx: adrenal insufficiency, allergies, RA, lupus, COPD

PREMARIN (conjugated estrogens): hormones, Rx: menopause

PREMPRO (estrogens/progesterone): hormones, Rx: menopause

PREVACID (lansoprazole): gastric acid pump inhibitor, Rx: ulcers, esophagitis, GERD

PREVPAC (lansoprazole/amoxicillin/clarithromycin): H. Pylori treatment, Rx: duodenal ulcers

PRIFTIN (rifapentine): antibiotic, Rx: tuberculosis

PRILOSEC (omeprazole): gastric acid pump inhibitor, Rx: ulcers, esophagitis, GERD

Primaquine: antimalarial agent, Rx: malaria

PRIMATENE MIST (epinephrine): alpha/beta agonist, Rx: bronchospasms, asthma

PRIMAXIN (imipenem/cilastatin): carbapenem antibiotic, Rx: bacterial infections

Primidone (MYSOLINE): anticonvulsant, Rx: seizures

PRINIVIL (lisinopril): ACE inhibitor, Rx: HTN, CHF

PRINZIDE (lisinopril/HCTZ): ACE inhibitor/diuretic, Rx: HTN

PRISTIQ (desvenlafaxine): antidepressant, Rx: depression

PROAMATINE (midodrine): vasopressor, Rx: orthostatic hypotension

PRO-BANTHINE (propantheline): anticholinergic, inhibits gastric acid secretion, Rx: peptic ulcers

Probenecid: increases uric acid secretion, Rx: gout

Procainamide (PROCANBID): antiarrhythmic, Rx: dysrhythmias

PROCANBID (procainamide): antiarrhythmic, Rx: dysrhythmias

Procarbazine (MATULANE): antineoplastic, Rx: Hodgkin's disease

PROCARDIA, PROCARDIA XL (nifedipine): calcium channel blocker, Rx: angina, HTN

Prochlorperazine (COMPAZINE): phenothiazine antiemetic, Rx: nausea and vomiting, anxiety

PROCRIT (epoetin alfa): stimulates red blood cell production, Rx: anemia, in renal failure, HIV, and chemotherapy

PROCTOCORT (hydrocortisone): rectal corticosteroid, Rx: ulcerative colitis

PROCTOFOAM-HC (hydrocortisone): steroid anti-inflammatory, Rx: inflammation, itching

Progesterone (PROMETRIUM): progestin, Rx: endometrial hyperplasia, secondary amenorrhea

PROGRAF (tacrolimus): immunosuppressant, Rx: transplant

PROLASTIN (alpha-1 proteinase inhibitor): Rx: alpha-1 antitrypsin deficiency, emphysema

Promethazine (PHENERGAN): phenothiazine, Rx: rhinitis, allergic conjunctivitis, sedation, nausea and vomiting

PROMETRIUM (progesterone): progestin, Rx: endometrial hyperplasia, secondary amenorrhea

Propafenone (RYTHMOL): beta blocker, antiarrhythmic, Rx: PSVT, paroxysmal atrial fibrillation

Propantheline: anticholinergic, inhibits gastric acid secretion, Rx: peptic ulcers

Proparacaine OPTH (ALCAINE): anesthetic, Rx: corneal anesthesia

PROPECIA (finasteride): 5-alpha-reductase inhibitor, Rx: hair loss, men only

Propoxyphene (DARVON): opioid analgesic, Rx: mild to moderate pain

Propoxyphene/APAP (DARVON): opioid analgesic, Rx: mild to moderate pain

Propranolol (INDERAL): beta blocker, Rx: HTN, prophylaxis of: angina, cardiac dysrhythmias, AMI, migraine headache

Propylthiouracil: antithyroid, Rx: hyperthyroidism

PROSCAR (finasteride): antiandrogen, Rx: benign prostatic hypertrophy

PROSED/DS (methenamine/phenyl salicylate/methylene blue/benzoic acid/hyoscyamine): bactericidal, analgesic, antiseptic, Rx: urinary tract infections

PROSOM (estazolam): benzodiazepine hypnotic, Rx: insomnia

PROTONIX (pantoprazole): proton pump inhibitor, Rx: ulcers, GERD

PROTOPAM (pralidoxime): anticholinergic, Rx: organophosphate poisoning

PROVENTIL, PROVENTIL HFA (albuterol): beta$_2$ agonist bronchodilator, Rx: COPD, asthma

PROVERA (medroxyprogesterone): hormone, Rx: amenorrhea, irregular vaginal bleeding

PROVIGIL (modafinil): stimulant, Rx: narcolepsy, daytime sleepiness

PROZAC (fluoxetine): a heterocyclic antidepressant

Pseudoephedrine (SUDAFED): decongestant, Rx: colds, allergies

Psyllium (KONSYL, METAMUCIL): fiber laxative, Rx: constipation

PULMICORT (budesonide): inhaled corticosteroid, Rx: asthma

PULMOZYME (dornase alfa): lytic enzyme, dissolves lung secretions, Rx: cystic fibrosis
PURINETHOL (mercaptopurine): antineplastic, Rx: leukemia
Pyrazinamide: antibacterial, Rx: tuberculosis
PYRIDIUM (phenazopyridine): urinary tract analgesic, Rx: relief of pain on urination
Pyridostigmine (MESTINON): anticholinesterase, Rx: myasthenia gravis
Pyridoxine (vitamin B6): vitamin
Pyrimethamine (DARAPRIM): antiparasitic, Rx: toxoplasmosis, malaria

Q

QUALAQUIN (quinine): antimalarial, Rx: malaria
QUESTRAN (cholestyramine): bile acid sequestrant, Rx: antihyperlipidemic
Quetiapine (SEROQUEL): antipsychotic, Rx: schizophrenia, bipolar disorder
Quinapril (ACCUPRIL): ACE inhibitor, Rx: HTN, CHF
Quinapril/HCTZ (QUINARETIC, ACCURETIC): ACE inhibitor/ diuretic, Rx: HTN
QUINARETIC (quinapril/HCTZ): ACE inhibitor/diuretic, Rx: HTN
Quinidine: antiarrhythmic, Rx: atrial fibrillation/flutter, malaria
Quinine: antimalarial, Rx: malaria
Quinupristin/Dalfopristin (SYNERCID): streptogramin antibiotic, Rx: bacterial infections
QUIXIN OPTH (levofloxacin): fluoroquinolone, Rx: conjunctivitis
QVAR (beclomethasone): inhaled corticosteroid, Rx: asthma

R

Raloxifene (EVISTA): estrogen modulator, Rx: osteoporosis, breast cancer prevention
Ramipril (ALTACE): ACE inhibitor, Rx: HTN, CHF post MI
RANEXA (ranolazine): anti-ischemic, Rx: chronic angina
Ranitidine (ZANTAC): histamine-2 blocker, Rx: ulcers, GERD, esophagitis
RAPAFLO (silodosin): alpha receptor agonist, Rx: benign prostatic hyperplasia

RAPAMUNE (sirolimus): immunosuppressive, Rx: renal transplant

RAPTIVA (efalizumab): immunosuppressant, Rx: psoriasis

RAZADYNE (galantamine): acetylcholinesterase inhibitor,
Rx: Alzheimer's disease

REBETOL (ribavirin): antiviral, Rx: hepatitis C

REBETRON (interferon alfa/ribavirin): antivirals, Rx: hepatitis C

Rebif (interferon-beta-1a): immunomodulator, Rx: multiple sclerosis

RECOMBINATE (Factor VIII): antihemophilic factor, Rx: hemophilia

REFLUDAN (lepirudin): anticoagulant, Rx: heparin induced
thrombocytopenia

REGLAN (metoclopramide): improves gastric emptying,
Rx: heartburn, diabetic gastroparesis

RELAFEN (nabumetone): NSAID analgesic, Rx: arthritis

RELENZA (zanamivir): antiviral, Rx: influenza

RELISTOR (methylnaltrexone): GI tract opioid antagonist,
Rx: opioid induced constipation

RELPAX (eletriptan): serotonin receptor agonist, Rx: migraine
headaches

REMERON (mirtazapine): antidepressant, Rx: depression

REMICADE (infliximab): neutralizes tumor necrosis factor,
Rx: Crohn's disease, arthritis, ulcerative colitis, psoriasis

RENAGEL (sevelamer): phosphate binder, Rx: hyperphosphatemia
in renal disease

REQUIP (ropinirole): dopaminergic, Rx: Parkinson's disease,
restless legs syndrome

RESCRIPTOR (delavirdine): antiretroviral, Rx: HIV

RESTASIS OPTH (cyclosporine): immunomodulator, Rx: increases
tear production

RESTORIL (temazepam): benzodiazepine hypnotic, Rx: insomnia

RETEVASE (reteplase): thrombolytic, Rx: AMI

RETIN A (tretinoin): retinoid, Rx: acne

RETROVIR (zidovudine): antiretroviral agent, Rx: HIV

REVATIO (sildenafil): vasodilator, Rx: pulmonary artery hypertension

REYATAZ (atazanavir): antiretroviral, Rx: HIV

RHINOCORT (budesonide): nasal corticosteroid, Rx: allergic rhinitis

Ribavirin (REBETOL): antiviral, Rx: hepatitis C

RIFADIN (rifampin): antibiotic, Rx: tuberculosis, prophylaxis for
N. meningitidis

RIFAMATE (rifampin/isoniazid): antibiotics, Rx: tuberculosis

Rifampin (RIFADIN): antibiotic, Rx: tuberculosis, prophylaxis for N. meningitidis

Rifapentine (PRIFTIN): antibiotic, Rx: tuberculosis

RIFATER (isoniazid/rifampin/pyrazinamide): antibiotic, Rx: tuberculosis

Rifaximin (XIFAXAN): antibiotic, Rx: traveler's diarrhea, hepatic encephalopathy

Rimantadine (FLUMADINE): antiviral, Rx: influenza A virus

RIOMET (metformin): oral hypoglycemic, Rx: diabetes (type 2)

Risedronate (ACTONEL): bone stabilizer, Rx: Paget's disease, osteoporosis

RISPERDAL (risperidone): antipsychotic, Rx: schizophrenia, autism, bipolar disorder

Risperidone (RISPERDAL): antipsychotic, Rx: schizophrenia, autism, bipolar disorder

RITALIN (methylphenidate): stimulant, Rx: attention deficit hyperactivity disorder in children, narcolepsy

Ritonavir (NORVIR): antiretroviral, Rx: HIV

RITUXAN (rituximab): antineoplastic, Rx: non-Hodgkin lymphoma, RA

Rivastigmine (EXELON): cholinesterase inhibitor, Rx: dementia in Alzheimer's disease and Parkinson's disease

ROBAXIN (methocarbamol): skeletal muscle relaxant

ROBINUL, ROBINUL FORTE (glycopyrrolate): anticholinergic, Rx: peptic ulcers

ROBITUSSIN (guaifenesin): expectorant

ROCALTROL (calcitrol): vitamin D analog, Rx: hypocalcemia in renal disease, hypoparathyroidism, bone disease

ROCEPHIN (ceftriaxone): cephalosporin antibiotic, Rx: bacterial infections

Ropinirole (REQUIP): dopaminergic, Rx: Parkinson's disease, restless leg syndrome

Rosiglitazone (AVANDIA): oral hypoglycemic, Rx: diabetes (type 2)

ROWASA (mesalamine): anti-inflammatory, Rx: colitis, proctitis

ROXANOL (morphine): opioid analgesic, Rx: moderate to severe pain

ROXICET (oxycodone/APAP): opioid analgesic, Rx: moderate to severe pain

ROXICODONE (oxycodone): opioid analgesic, Rx: moderate to severe pain

ROZEREM (ramelteon): melatonin agonist, Rx: insomnia

RYNATAN (phenylephrine/chlorpheniramine/pyrilamine): antihistamine/decongestant compound, Rx: common cold
RYNATUSS: antitussive/decongestant/antihistamine, Rx: common cold
RYTHMOL, RYTHMOL SR (propafenone): antiarrhythmic, Rx: PSVT, paroxysmal atrial fibrillation

S

SALAGEN (pilocarpine): cholinergic, Rx: dry mouth
SALIVART: saliva substitute, Rx: dry mouth
Salmeterol (SEREVENT): inhaled beta$_2$ bronchodilator, Rx: asthma, COPD
SAL-PLANT Gel (salicylic acid): for removal of common warts
Salsalate: NSAID analgesic, Rx: arthritis
SANDIMMUNE (cyclosporine): immunosuppressant agent, Rx: organ transplants
SANDOSTATIN (octreotide): antidiarrheal, growth inhibitor, Rx: acromegaly, diarrhea associated with carcinoid and intestinal tumors
Saquinavir (INVIRASE): antiretroviral, Rx: HIV
SARAFEM (fluoxetine): antidepressant, Rx: premenstrual dysphoric disorder
SAVELLA (milnacipran): selective serotonin/norepinephrine inhibitor, Rx: fibromyalgia
Scopolamine: anticholinergic, Rx: motion sickness, IBS, diverticulitis
SECONAL (secobarbital): barbiturate hypnotic, Rx: insomnia
SECTRAL (acebutolol): beta blocker, Rx: HTN, angina, dysrhythmias
Selegiline (ELDEPRYL): MAO inhibitor, Rx: Parkinson's disease
SEMPREX-D (acrivastine/pseudoephedrine): antihistamine/decongestant, Rx: allergic rhinitis
Senna Extract (SENOKOT): laxative, Rx: constipation
SENNA-S, SENOKOT-S (senna/docusate): laxative/stool softener, Rx: constipation
SENOKOT, SENOKOT XTRA (senna): laxative, Rx: constipation
SENSIPAR (cinacalcet): reduces PTH levels, Rx: 2nd hyperparathyroidism in dialysis patients
SEPTRA, SEPTRA DS (trimethoprim/sulfamethoxazole): sulfa antibacterial compound, Rx: bacterial infections

SEREVENT (salmeterol): inhaled beta$_2$ bronchodilator, Rx: asthma, COPD

SEROQUEL (quetiapine): antipsychotic, Rx: schizophrenia, bipolar disorder

SEROSTIM (somatropin): hormone, Rx: AIDS wasting

Sertraline (ZOLOFT): antidepressant, Rx: depression, panic disorder, obsessive-compulsive disorder, premenstrual dysphoric disorder

SERZONE (nefazodone): antidepressant, Rx: depression

SIMCOR (niacin/simvastatin): cholesterol reducers, Rx: hypercholesterolemia, hypertriglyceridemia

Simethicone (MYLICON): Rx: relief of excess gas in GI tract

SIMPLY COUGH LIQUID (dextromethorphan): antitussive, Rx: cough

Simvastatin (Zocor): statin, Rx: hypercholesterolemia, CAD

SINEMET CR (carbidopa/levodopa): dopamine precursors, Rx: Parkinson's disease

SINEQUAN (doxepin): tricyclic antidepressant, Rx: depression, anxiety

SINGULAIR (montelukast): leukotriene receptor antagonist, Rx: asthma, allergic rhinitis

SINUVENT (phenylephrine/guaifenesin): decongestant/ expectorant, Rx: sinusitis, rhinitis

Sirolimus (RAPAMUNE): immunosuppressive, Rx: renal transplant

SKELAXIN (metaxalone): skeletal muscle relaxant

SLO-NIACIN (niacin CR): Rx: hypercholesterolemia, hypertriglyceridemia

Sodium polysterene sulfonate (KAYEXALATE): Na/K exchange resin, Rx: hyperkalemia

SOMA (carisoprodol): muscle relaxant, Rx: muscle spasm

SONATA (zaleplon): hypnotic, Rx: insomnia

SORIATANE (acitretin): retinoid, Rx: psoriasis

Sotalol (BETAPACE): antiarrhythmic, Rx: dysrhythmias

SPECTRACEF (cefditoren): cephalosporin antibiotic, Rx: bacterial infections

SPIRIVA (tiotropium): inhaled anticholinergic bronchodilator, Rx: COPD

Spironolactone (ALDACTONE): potassium-sparing diuretic, Rx: hyperaldosteronism, HTN, CHF

SPORANOX (itraconazole): antifungal, Rx: fungal infections

SSKI (potassium iodide): expectorant, Rx: asthma, bronchitis

STADOL NS (butorphanol): opioid agonist/antagonist analgesic, Rx: pain

STAGESIC (hydrocodone and acetaminophen): analgesic combination (opioid), Rx: pain

STALEVO (levodopa/carbidopa/entacapone): dopamine precursors, Rx: Parkinson's disease

STARLIX (nateglinide): oral hypoglycemic, Rx: diabetes (type 2)

STATUSS DM (dextromethorphan, phenylephrine, chlorpheniramine): non-narcotic antitussive, decongestant, antihistamine compound

Stavudine d4T (ZERIT): antiretroviral, Rx: HIV

STELAZINE (trifluoperazine): antipsychotic, Rx: schizophrenia

STRATTERA (atomoxetine): psychotherapeutic agent, Rx: ADHD

Streptomycin: aminoglycoside antibiotic, Rx: tuberculosis

STRIANT (testosterone): androgen, Rx: adult male hypogonadism

STROMECTOL (ivermectin): anti-parasite, Rx: intestinal nematodes

SUBOXONE (buprenorphine/naloxone): opioid analgesic/antagonist, Rx: opiate addiction

SUBUTEX (buprenorphine): narcotic analgesic, Rx: opiate addiction

Sucralfate (CARAFATE): anti-ulcer agent, Rx: duodenal ulcers

Sufentanil (SUFENTA): analgesic, opioid, general anesthetic, Rx: analgesic supplement

SULAR (nisoldipine): calcium channel blocker, Rx: HTN

Sulfacetamide OPTH (BLEPH-10): antibiotic, Rx: ocular infections

Sulfamethoxazole (SEPTRA): sulfa antibiotic, Rx: bacterial infections

Sulfasalazine (AZULFIDINE): anti-inflammatory, Rx: ulcerative colitis, rheumatoid arthritis

Sulfisoxazole (GANTRISIN): sulfonamide antibiotic, Rx: bacterial infections

Sulindac (CLINORIL): NSAID analgesic, Rx: arthritis

Sumatriptan (IMITREX): selective serotonin receptor agonist, Rx: migraine headache

SUPRAX (cefixime): cephalosporin antibiotic, Rx: bacterial infections

SURVANTA (beractant): lung surfactant in premature infants

SUSTIVA (efavirenz): antiretroviral, Rx: HIV

SYMBICORT (budesonide/formoterol): inhaled corticosteroid/beta$_2$ agonist, Rx: asthma, COPD

SYMBYAX (olanzapine/fluoxetine): antipsychotic/SSRI, Rx: bipolar disorder, resistant depression

SYMMETREL (amantadine): antiparkinson/antiviral, Rx: influenza A, Parkinson's disease

SYNAGIS (palivizumab): antiviral antibody, Rx: respiratory syncytial virus (prevention)
SYNAREL (naferelin): nasal gonadotropin-releasing hormone, Rx: endometriosis, precocious puberty
SYNERCID (quinupristin/dalfopristin): streptogramin antibiotic, Rx: bacterial infections
SYNTHROID (levothyroxine): thyroid hormone, Rx: hypothyroidism

T

TABLOID (thioguanine): antineoplastic, Rx: leukemia
TAGAMET (cimetidine): inhibits gastric acid secretion, Rx: ulcers
TALACEN (pentazocine/APAP): opioid agonist/antagonist analgesic/APAP, Rx: pain
TALWIN NX (pentazocine/naloxone): opioid agonist/antagonist analgesic, Rx: pain
TAMBOCOR (flecainide): antiarrhythmic, Rx: PSVT, paroxysmal atrial fibrillation
TAMIFLU (oseltamivir): antiviral, Rx: influenza
Tamoxifen: antiestrogen, Rx: breast cancer
TAPAZOLE (methimazole): antithyroid, Rx: hyperthyroidism
TARKA (trandolapril/verapamil): ACE inhibitor/calcium channel blocker, Rx: HTN
TASMAR (tolcapone): antiparkinson agent, COMT inhibitor, Rx: Parkinson's disease
TEGRETOL, TEGRETOL XR (carbamazepine): anticonvulsant, Rx: seizures, trigeminal neuralgia
TEKTURNA (Aliskeren): direct renin inhibitor, Rx: HTN
Telmisartan (MICARDIS): angiotensin II receptor agonist, Rx: HTN
Temazepam (RESTORIL): benzodiazepine hypnotic, Rx: insomnia
TENEX (guanfacine): centrally acting alpha agonist, Rx: HTN
TENORETIC (atenolol/Chlorthalidone): beta blocker/diuretic, Rx: HTN
TENORMIN (atenolol): beta blocker, Rx: hypertension, angina, MI
TENUATE (diethylpropion): stimulant, appetite suppressant, Rx: obesity
Terazosin (HYTRIN): alpha-1 blocker, Rx: HTN, benign prostatatic hyperplasia
Terbinafine (LAMISIL): antifungal, Rx: nail fungus, ringworm
Terbutaline (BRETHINE): beta$_2$ agonist bronchodilator, Rx: asthma, COPD

TESSALON (benzonatate): antitussive, Rx: cough
Testosterone (ANDRODERM, DEPO-TESTOSTERONE):
androgen, Rx: hypogonadism
TESTRED (methyltestosterone): androgen, Rx: hypogonadism
Tetracycline (SUMYCIN): tetracycline antibiotic, Rx: bacterial
infections
TEVETEN (eprosartan): angiotensin II receptor inhibitor, Rx: HTN
Thalidomide (THALOMID): immunosuppressant, Rx: HIV, leprosy
THALOMID (thalidomide): immunosuppressant, Rx: HIV, leprosy
THEO-24 (theophylline): bronchodilator, Rx: asthma, COPD
THEOCRON (theophylline): bronchodilator, Rx: asthma, COPD
Theophylline (THEO-24, UNIPHYL): bronchodilator, Rx: asthma,
COPD
Thiamin: vitamin B1, Rx: thiamin deficiency
Thioridazine: antipsychotic, Rx: schizophrenia
Thiothixene (NAVANE): antipsychotic, Rx: schizophrenia
THORAZINE (chlorpromazine): antipsychotic, Rx: schizophrenia
Thyroid (ARMOUR THYROID): thyroid hormone,
Rx: hypothyroidism
THYROLAR (liotrix): thyroid hormone, Rx: hypothyroidism
Tiagabine (GABITRIL): anticonvulsant, Rx: partial seizures
TIAZAC (diltiazem): calcium channel blocker, Rx: HTN, angina
Ticarcillin/clavulanate (TIMENTIN): penicillin antibiotic,
Rx: bacterial infections
TICLID (ticlopidine): platelet inhibitor, Rx: stroke prophylaxis
Ticlodipine (TICLID): platelet inhibitor, Rx: stroke prophylaxis
TIGAN (trimethobenzamide): antiemetic, Rx: postoperative nausea
and vomiting
TIKOSYN (dofetilide): antiarrhythmic, Rx: atrial fibrillation
TIMENTIN (ticarcillin/clavulanate): penicillin class antibiotic,
Rx: bacterial infections
Timolol (BLOCADREN): beta blocker, Rx: HTN, MI, migraine
TIMOPTIC OPTH (timolol): beta blocker, Rx: glaucoma
Tizanidine (ZANAFLEX): skeletal muscle relaxant
TOBI Solution Inhalation (tobramycin): aminoglycoside antibiotic,
Rx: cystic fibrosis
TOBRADEX (tobramycin/dexamethasone): antibiotic/steroid,
Rx: eye infection/inflammation
Tobramycin: aminoglycoside antibiotic, Rx: bacterial infections
TOBREX OPTH (tobramycin): aminoglycoside antibiotic,
Rx: ocular infections

TOFRANIL, TOFRANIL PM (imipramine): tricyclic antidepressant, Rx: depression, anxiety

Tolazamide: oral hypoglycemic, Rx: diabetes (type 2)

Tolbutamide: oral hypoglycemic, Rx: diabetes (type 2)

Tolmetin: NSAID analgesic, Rx: arthritis

Tolterodine (DETROL): urinary bladder antispasmodic, Rx: overactive bladder

TOPAMAX (topiramate): anticonvulsant, Rx: seizures, migraine

TOPROL-XL (metoprolol): cardioselective beta blocker, Rx: HTN, angina, CHF

TORADOL (ketorolac): NSAID analgesic, Rx: acute pain

Torsemide (DEMADEX): loop diuretic, Rx: HTN, edema in CHF, kidney disease, liver disease

TOVIAZ (fesoterodine): anticholinergic, Rx: overactive bladder

TRACLEER (bosentan): endothelin receptor antagonist, Rx: pulmonary hypertension

Tramadol (ULTRAM): opioid analgesic, Rx: moderate to severe pain

TRANDATE (labetalol): beta blocker, Rx: hypertension

Trandolapril (MAVIK): ACE inhibitor, Rx: HTN, CHF post MI

TRANSDERM-SCOP (scopolamine): anticholinergic antiemetic, Rx: motion sickness prophylaxis

TRANXENE (clorazepate): benzodiazepine hypnotic, Rx: anxiety, seizures

TRAVATAN OPTH (travoprost): prostaglandin agonist, Rx: glaucoma

Trazodone: antidepressant, Rx: depression, insomnia

TRECATOR (ethionamide): antibiotic, Rx: tuberculosis

TRENTAL (pentoxifylline): reduces blood viscosity, Rx: intermittent claudication

Triamcinolone (AZMACORT): inhaled corticosteroid, Rx: asthma

Triamterene/HCTZ (DYAZIDE, Maxzide): diuretics, Rx: HTN, water retention

Triazolam (HALCION): benzodiazepine hypnotic, Rx: insomnia

TRICOR (fenofibrate): lipid regulator, Rx: hyperlipidemia

Trifluoperazine (STELAZINE): antipsychotic, Rx: schizophrenia

TRIGLIDE (fenofibrate): lipid reducer, Rx: hyperlipidemia

Trihexyphenidyl (ARTANE): anticholinergic, Rx: Parkinson's disease

TRILEPTAL (oxcarbazepine): anticonvulsant, Rx: partial seizures

Trimethoprim: antibiotic, Rx: UTI

Trimethoprim/Sulfamethoxazole (BACTRIM, SEPTRA): sulfa antibiotic compound, Rx: bacterial infections

TRINESSA (ethinyl estradiol and norgestimate): contraceptive, Rx: prevent pregnancy, acne

TRI-NORINYL (ethinyl estradiol and norethindrone): contraceptive, Rx: prevent pregnancy, acne, menopause

TRIPHASIL (ethinyl estradiol and levonorgestrel): contraceptive, Rx: prevent pregnancy

TRIZIVIR (abacavir/lamivudine/zidovudine): antiretrovirals, Rx: HIV infection, hepatitis B

TRUSOPT OPTH (dorzolamide): decreases intraocular pressure Rx: glaucoma

TRUVADA (emtricitabine/tenofovir): antiretrovirals, Rx: HIV

TUSSAFED HC (hydrocodone/phenylephrine/guaifenesin): opioid antitussive/decongestant/expectorant

TUSSI-ORGANIDIN (guaifenesin/codeine): expectorant/opioid antitussive, Rx: cough

TUSSIONEX (hydrocodone/chlorpheniramine): opioid antitussive/antihistamine, Rx: coughs, allergies, cold

TYGACIL (tigecycline): glycylcycline antibiotic, Rx: bacterial infections

TYKERB (lapatinib): antineoplastic agent, Rx: breast cancer

TYLENOL w/Codeine (APAP, codeine): opioid with APAP analgesic, Rx: mild to moderate pain

TYLENOL SINUS CONGESTION (phenylephrine/guaifenesin/APAP): decongestant/expectorant/analgesic, Rx: sinusitis, rhinitis, colds

TYZEKA (telbivudine): antiviral, Rx: hepatitis B

U

ULORIC (febuxostat): xanthine oxidase inhibitor, Rx: gout

ULTRACET (tramadol/APAP): opioid analgesic compound, Rx: acute pain

ULTRAM (tramadol): opioid analgesic, Rx: moderate to severe pain

ULTRASE, ULTRASE MT (pancrelipase): pancreatic enzymes replacement, Rx: chronic pancreatitis, cystic fibrosis

UNIPHYL (theophylline): bronchodilator, Rx: asthma, COPD

UNIRETIC (moexipril/HCTZ): ACE inhibitor/diuretic, Rx: HTN

UNISOM (doxylamine): antihistamine sedative, Rx: insomnia

UNIVASC (moexipril): ACE inhibitor, Rx: HTN

URECHOLINE (bethanechol): cholinergic, Rx: urinary retention

URIMAX (methenamine/salicylate/methylene blue/hyoscyamine): bactericidal, analgesic, antispasmodic, Rx: urinary tract infections
UROXATRAL (alfuzosin): smooth muscle relaxant, Rx: BPH
UROCIT-K (potassium citrate): urinary alkalinizer, Rx: kidney stones
Ursodiol (ACTIGALL): bile acid, Rx: gallstones

V

Valacyclovir (VALTREX): antiviral, Rx: herpes, shingles
VALCYTE (valganciclovir): antiviral, Rx: cytomegalovirus
VALIUM (diazepam): benzodiazepine hypnotic, Rx: anxiety, muscle spasms, seizures, alcohol withdrawal
Valproic acid (DEPAKENE): anticonvulsant, Rx: seizures, migraines, mania
Valrubicin (VALSTAR): antineoplastic, Rx: bladder cancer
Valsartan (DIOVAN): angiotensin II receptor inhibitor, Rx: HTN, CHF, post-MI
VALTREX (valacyclovir): antiviral, Rx: herpes, shingles
VANCOCIN (vancomycin): antibiotic, Rx: bacterial infections
Vancomycin (VANCOCIN): antibiotic, Rx: bacterial infections
VANTIN (cefpodoxime): cephalosporin antibiotic, Rx: bacterial infections
VAPRISOL (conivaptan): increased water excretion, Rx: hyponatremia
VASERETIC (enalapril/HCTZ): ACE inhibitor/diuretic, Rx: HTN
VECTIBIX (panitumamab): antineoplastic, Rx: colorectal cancer
VASOTEC (enalaprilat): ACE inhibitor, Rx: HTN, CHF
VECTIBIX (panitumamab): antineoplastic, Rx: colorectal cancer
Venlafaxine (EFFEXOR): antidepressant, Rx: depression, anxiety, panic disorder
VENOFER (iron sucrose): Rx: iron deficiency anemia in chronic kidney disease and dialysis
VENTOLIN (albuterol): beta$_2$ agonist bronchodilator, Rx: asthma, COPD
Verapamil (CALAN, COVERA-HS, ISOPTIN): calcium channel blocker, Rx: angina, PSVT, HTN
VERELAN, VERELAN PM (verapamil): calcium blocker, Rx: angina, hypertension, PSVT

VERMOX (mebendazole): anthelminthic, Rx: intestinal worms
VESICARE (solifenacin): anticholinergic, Rx: overactive bladder
VFEND (voriconazole): antifungal, Rx: fungal infections
VIAGRA (sildenafil): vasodialator, Rx: male erectile dysfunction
VIBRAMYCIN (doxycycline): tetracycline antibiotic, Rx: bacterial infections
VICODIN, VICODIN ES (hydrocodone/APAP): narcotic analgesic compound, Rx: moderate to severe pain
VIDEX (didanosine): antiretroviral, Rx: HIV
VIGAMOX OPTH (moxifloxacin): fluoroquinolone antibiotic, Rx: bacterial conjunctivitis
VIMPAT (lacosamide): anticonvulsant, Rx: partial onset seizure
VIOKASE (pancrelipase): pancreatic enzymes replacement, Rx: chronic pancreatitis, cystic fibrosis
VIRACEPT (nelfinavir): antiretroviral, Rx: HIV
VIRAMUNE (nevirapine): antiretroviral, Rx: HIV
VIREAD (tenofovir): antiretroviral, Rx: HIV, hepatitis B
VISKEN (pindolol): beta blocker, Rx: HTN
VISTARIL (hydroxyzine): antihistamine, Rx: pruritis, sedation, anxiety
VIVELLE (estradiol): transdermal estrogen, Rx: symptoms of menopause
VOLTAREN (diclofenac): NSAID analgesic, Rx: arthritis, pain
VYTORIN (ezetimibe/simvastatin): antihyperlipidemics, Rx: high cholesterol

W

Warfarin (COUMADIN): anticoagulant, Rx: A-Fib, thrombosis
WELCHOL (colesevelam): bile acid sequestrant, Rx: hyperlipidemia
WELLBUTRIN (bupropion): antidepressant, Rx: depression

X

XALATAN OPTH (latanoprost): reduces intraocular pressure, Rx: glaucoma
XANAX, XANAX XR (alprazolam): benzodiazepine, Rx: anxiety disorder, panic attacks
XELODA (capecitabine): antineoplastic, Rx: breast cancer, colorectal cancer

XENICAL (orlistat): lipase inhibitor, Rx: obesity
XIFAXAN (rifaximin): antibiotic, Rx: traveler's diarrhea, hepatic encephalopathy
XOPENEX (levalbuterol): inhaled beta$_2$ bronchodilator, Rx: asthma, COPD

Y

YASMIN 28 (drospirenone/estradiol): oral contraceptive
YAZ (drospirenone/estradiol): oral contraceptive
YODOXIN (iodoquinol): amebicide, Rx: intestinal amebiasis

Z

ZADITOR OPTH (ketotifen): antihistamine, Rx: allergic conjunctivitis
Zaleplon (SONATA): hypnotic, Rx: insomnia
ZANAFLEX (tizanidine): skeletal muscle relaxant
ZARONTIN (ethosuximide): anticonvulsant, Rx: absence seizure
ZAROXOLYN (metolazone): thiazide diuretic, Rx: HTN, fluid retention
ZEBETA (bisoprolol): beta blocker, Rx: HTN
ZEGERID (omeprazole/sodium bicarbonate): proton pump inhibitor compound, Rx: stress ulcer, ulcers, GERD
ZEMPLAR (paricalcitol): vitamin D analog, Rx: hyperparathyroidism in chronic kidney disease
ZERIT (stavudine d4T): antiretroviral, Rx: HIV
ZESTORETIC (lisinopril/HCTZ): ACE inhibitor/diuretic, Rx: HTN
ZESTRIL (lisinopril): ACE inhibitor, Rx: HTN, CHF
ZETIA (ezetimibe): antihyperlipidemic, Rx: hypercholesterolemia
ZIAC (bisoprolol/HCTZ): beta blocker/diuretic, Rx: HTN
ZIAGEN (abacavir): antiretroviral, Rx: HIV
Zidovudine (AZT, RETROVIR): antiretroviral, Rx: HIV
ZINACEF (cefuroxime): cephalosporin antibiotic, Rx: bacterial infections
ZINECARD (dexrazoxane): cardioprotective agent, chelating agent, Rx: cardiomyopathy caused by doxorubicin
ZITHROMAX (azithromycin): macrolide antibiotic, Rx: bacterial infections
ZOCOR (simvastatin): statin, Rx: hypercholesterolemia, CAD

ZOFRAN (ondansetron): 5-HT3 receptor agonist, Rx: nausea and vomiting due to chemotherapy, radiation, and surgery

ZOLADEX (goserelin): gonadotropin-releasing hormone agonist, Rx: endometriosis, prostate cancer, breast cancer

ZOLOFT (sertraline): antidepressant, Rx: depression, OCD, social anxiety disorder

Zolpidem (AMBIEM): hypnotic, Rx: insomnia

ZOMETA (zoledronic acid): biphosphonate, Rx: hypercalcemia of malignancy

ZOMIG (zolmitriptan): serotonin receptor agonist, Rx: migraine headache

ZONEGRAN (zonisamide): anticonvulsant, Rx: partial seizures

Zonisamide (ZONEGRAN): anticonvulsant, Rx: partial seizures

ZOSYN (piperacillin/tazobactam): penicillin class antibiotic, Rx: bacterial infections

ZOVIRAX (acyclovir): antiviral, Rx: herpes, shingles, chickenpox

ZYBAN (buproprion): antidepressant, Rx: smoking cessation

ZYFLO (zileuton): bronchospasm inhibitor, Rx: asthma

ZYLOPRIM (allopurinol): xanthine oxidase inhibitor, Rx: gout

ZYMAR OPTH (gatifloxacin): fluoroquinolone, Rx: bacterial conjunctivitis

ZYPREXA, ZYPREXA ZYDIS (olanzapine) antipsychotic, Rx: schizophrenia, bipolar disorder

ZYRTEC (cetirizine): antihistamine, Rx: allergy, hives, asthma

ZYRTEC D (cetirizine/pseudoephedrine): antihistamine/decongestant, Rx: allergic rhinitis

ZYVOX (linezolid): oxazolidinone antibiotic, Rx: bacterial infections

Drugs

Abbreviations

1°	primary, first degree	$\overline{c}$	with
2°	secondary, second degree	c/o	complaining of
3°	tertiary, third degree	CA	cancer
≤	less than; less than or equal to	CAO	conscious, alert, oriented
≥	greater than; greater than or equal to	CBG	capillary blood glucose
≡	approximately equal to	CHF	congestive heart failure
α	alpha	COPD	chronic obstructive pulmonary disease
$\overline{a}$	before	CPAP	continuous positive airway pressure
abd	abdomen	CVA	cerebrovascular accident (stroke)
ACE	angiotensin-converting enzyme	cx	chest
ADD	attention deficit disorder	D_5W	dextrose 5% in water
ADHD	attention deficit/ hyperactivity disorder	DIC	disseminated intravascular coagulation
AIDS	acquired immune deficiency syndrome	dL	deciliter (1/10 of 1 liter; 100 mL)
AMI	acute myocardial infarction	DMARD	disease-modifying antirheumatic drug
APAP	acetaminophen	DOE	dyspnea on exertion
APE	acute pulmonary edema	DSD	dry sterile dressing
ARC	AIDS related complex	Dx	diagnosis
ASA	acetylsalicylic acid (aspirin)	ECG	electrocardiogram
β	beta	ED	emergency

EPS	extra pyramidal symptoms (dystonias, akathisia, etc.)	IM	intramuscular
ETCO$_2$	end-tidal carbon dioxide	IO	intraosseous
Fem ♀	female	*IU	*unapproved abbreviation: write out "International Units"
FV	fever	IV	intravenous
Fx	fracture	IVP	IV push
g, gm	gram	IVR	idioventricular rhythm
GCS	Glasgow Coma Scale	K+	potassium ion
GI	gastrointestinal	KCl	potassium chloride
gr	grain	kg	kilogram (1,000 grams; 2.2 pounds)
gtt	drop	KVO	keep vein open (8 - 15 mL/hour)
GU	genitourinary	L	liter
H/A	headache	LOC	level of consciousness
HCTZ	hydrochlorothiazide	LP	lumbar puncture
HIV	human immuno-deficiency virus	LUQ	left upper quadrant
H&P	history and physical examintion	min	minute(s)
HR	heart rate	M ♂	male
HTN	hypertension	MAOI	monoamine oxidase inhibitor
Hx	history	mcg	microgram (1/1,000,000 of 1 gram)
ICP	intracranial pressure	MDI	metered dose inhaler
IJR	idiojunctional rhythm	mEq	milliequivalent
IL	intralingual	mg	milligram (1/1,000 of 1 gram)

MI	myocardial infarction	PR	per rectum; rectally
mL	milliliter (1/1,000 of 1 liter; 1 mL)	PSVT	paroxysmal supra-ventricular tachycardia
~~ms~~	write out morphine	PVC	premature ventricular contraction
~~MSO$_4$~~	write out morphine sulfate	q̄	every
NaHCO$_3$	sodium bicarbonate	RL	Ringer's lactate
N&V, N/V	nausea and vomiting	RR	respiratory rate
NAD	no acute distress, no apparent distress	Rx	prescribed for, used for
NG	nasogastric	s̄	without
NR	Normosol–R	s/s	signs and symptoms
NS	normal saline (0.9% NaCl)	SaO$_2$	arterial oxygen saturation
NSAID	non-steroidal anti-inflammatory drug	ScvO2	central venous oxygen saturation
NTG	nitroglycerin	SL	sublingual
OLMC	On-Line Medical Control	SOB	shortness of breath, dyspnea
p̄	after	SQ	subcutaneous
PCP	pneumocystis carinii	SW	sterile water
PETCO$_2$	partial pressure of end-tidal carbon dioxide	Sz	seizure
PO	by mouth, orally	TB	tuberculosis
POC	position of comfort	TCA	tricyclic antidepressant
prn	as needed	TKO	to keep open (8-15 mL/hour)

Torr	millimeters mercury (mm Hg)	WPW	Wolff-Parkinson-White (syndrome)
U	*write out "unit"	x	times
URI	upper respiratory infection	↓	decreased
UTI	urinary tract infection	↑	increased
UV	umbilical vein, ultraviolet	μ	micro (1/1,000,000)
VF	ventricular fibrillation	Δ	change (delta)
VNS	vagus nerve stimulator	⊘	no, none, null
VT	ventricular tachycardia		

Notes

Phone Numbers

911 Communications Center

American Red Cross

Chemtrec Emergency # 1-800-424-9300

Chemtrec Non-emergency # 1-800-262-8200

Children's Services

CISD Team

Crisis Center

Domestic Violence Shelter

HazMat Team

Homeless Shelter

Medical Examiner/Coroner

Medical Resource Hospital

National Response Center # 1-800-424-8802

Poison Control Center # 1-800-222-1222

Public Health Department

Sexual Abuse/Rape Victim Hotline

State/County EMS Office

Translation Services

Trauma Center

Other

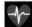

Heart Rate

First R wave

(measure to next R wave)

1500
750
500
375
300
250
214
187
167
150
136
125
115
107
100
94
88
83
79
75
71
68
65
63
60
58
56
54
52
50
48
47
46
45
44
43
42
41
40
39
38
37
36
35
34
33
32
31
30
27
25
23
21
20
19
18
17
16
15

CM.

PR Interval — .12 sec Min. / .20 sec Max.

QRS Width — .08 sec Min. / .12 sec Max.

QT Interval — .30 sec min. / .52 sec maximum

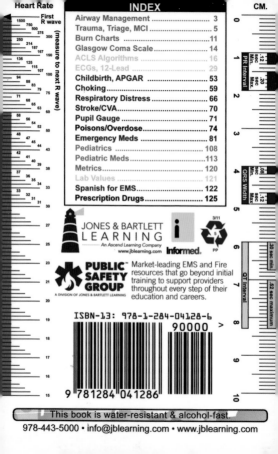

JONES & BARTLETT LEARNING
An Ascend Learning Company
www.jblearning.com

Informed.

3/11
PP

PUBLIC SAFETY GROUP™
A DIVISION OF JONES & BARTLETT LEARNING

Market-leading EMS and Fire resources that go beyond initial training to support providers throughout every step of their education and careers.

ISBN-13: 978-1-284-04128-6

90000 >

9 781284 041286

This book is water-resistant & alcohol-fast.

978-443-5000 • info@jblearning.com • www.jblearning.com